When Peter Payne, hero of *The Diary of a Teenage Health Freak*, was busy informing the world of his worries about acne and the length of certain parts of the anatomy, little did he realize that he had competition.

The competition is from Susie Payne – Pete's younger sister, but now an experienced sixteen-year-old, hoping to emulate her brother and even to outdo him. She writes about sex, romance, anorexia, glandular fever, depression, death, AIDS, dieting, taking exams, animal rights, contraception, divorce, worms, coping with stress, headlice, and many things besides. In her diary she not only includes cuttings, leaflets, letters, and other bits and pieces about the problems that concern her, but also records Pete Payne's continuing adventures and the events – both funny and sad – of their family life. Based as it is on carefully researched medical facts, her diary provides absolutely up-to-date information which will inform and entertain Susie's and Pete's contemporaries, teachers, and parents alike.

Ann McPherson and Aidan Macfarlane are both doctors working in Oxfordshire. They wrote the runaway best seller *The Diary of a Teenage Health Freak*, as well as *Mum, I Feel Funny*, which won the *Times Educational Supplement* Information Book Award. They have continued to carry out research into school health problems through questionnaires and talking to teenagers.

Ann McPherson is a General Practitioner with extensive experience of child health problems, both with her own children and with her patients. She is author of *Women's Problems in General Practice* and, with Ann Oakley and Helen Roberts, of *Miscarriage*.

Aidan Macfarlane is a Consultant Community Paediatrician with special interest in school health, who has also written *The Psychology of Childbirth* and *A Pocket Consultant in Child Health*.

John Astrop has written and illustrated many children's books, including *My Secret File, Not Now Dear!, After All We've Done!*, and *Ghastly Games*.

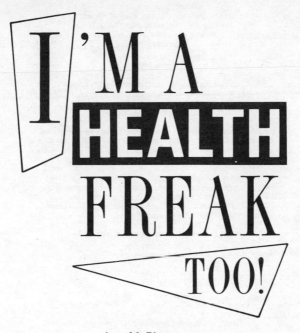

I'M A HEALTH FREAK TOO!

Ann McPherson
and
Aidan Macfarlane

Illustrated by
John Astrop

Oxford   New York

OXFORD UNIVERSITY PRESS

Oxford University Press, Walton Street, Oxford OX2 6DP

Oxford New York Toronto
Delhi Bombay Calcutta Madras Karachi
Petaling Jaya Singapore Hong Kong Tokyo
Nairobi Dar es Salaam Cape Town
Melbourne Auckland

and associated companies in
Berlin Ibadan

Oxford is a trade mark of Oxford University Press

British Library Cataloguing in Publication data
McPherson, Ann
I'm a health freak too!
1. Women. Health
I. Title II. Macfarlane, Aidan
613'.04244
ISBN 0–19–217769–9
ISBN 0–19–282232–2 Pbk

Library of Congress Cataloging in Publication Data
McPherson, Ann.
I'm a health freak too! / Ann McPherson, Aidan Macfarlane; illustrated by John Astrop.
p. cm.
Summary: A sixteen-year-old English girl writes in her diary about all the problems and events
of her life, which include romance, depression, animal rights, stress, and health.
[1. England—Fiction. 2. Diaries.] I. Macfarlane, Aidan, 1939–
II. Astrop, John, ill. III. Title.
Fic—dc19 PZ7.M478819 Iad 1989 89–31732
ISBN 0–19–217769–9
ISBN 0–19–282232–2 (pbk.)

Printed in Great Britain by
Richard Clay Ltd.
Bungay, Suffolk

Acknowledgements

Susie's diary is a combination of a large number of different voices and sources. We advertised in *Just Seventeen* and were overwhelmed by the avalanche of pale pink and yellow envelopes that snowed through the letter-box full of wonderful, and sometimes libellous, material. Three local upper schools in Oxfordshire—Peers, Lord Williams, and Cheney—once again put up with us invading the privacy of their pupils' lives with a detailed questionnaire on AIDS. Some of our children were more enthusiastic than others at contributing this time—Beth, Tamara and Tess, along with Gus, greatly helped in writing parts of it and casting more than a critical eye on the manuscript. Sam and Magnus were notable for their consistent reluctance to reveal any part of their teenage existence, while enjoying the fruits of the first book. For this we can only respect them. Among their many friends who helped us we would particularly like to acknowledge Amanda, Louise, Kitty, Gina and Matthew. Marney Leech advised us throughout and edited the final manuscript, as well as making numerous adjustments to avoid such errors as Easter Sunday occurring on a Friday. Jill Challner very kindly gave us the tables we use on pages 125-6. We were also helped by Ann Jeavons, Adèle Greene, Dick Mayon-White, Peter Morris, David Weatherall, Harriet Sansom, Mary Marzillier, Colin Blakemore, Richard Peto and John Galway. We are grateful to the Family Planning Association for providing the leaflet which forms the basis of pp 58-61.

To all these people, and the many others who have helped us in the preparation of both books, we would like to say THANK YOU.

Ann McPherson and Aidan Macfarlane

28 January 1989

Contents

PLAN OF MA FAMILLE

ADAM & EVE + SNAKE + APPLE

ATOMS

AMOEBAS

FISH

MONKEYS

Grandma Margret Portley (a *real* Granny – has false teeth) = Grandad Peter Portley (dead – run over by a car)

Grandma Daphne Payne (died cancer) = Grandad Tim Payne (died heart attack)

Uncle Bob (lost his prostate) = Aunt Pam (smells & loves kissing)

No children

Jane Elspeth Margret (Mum)

Aunt Jo = Uncle Geoff (tank driver in army)

Daisy

Paul (wets bed)

Anthony Tobias (Dad)

a baby brother who died at birth

PETE
Author of 'Diary of a Teenage Health Freak'

ME

SALLY
Lots of boyfriends and works in a pub

My cat Bovril's Family Tree

Bovril

Ginger Tom

5 kittens

Black Tom

2 kittens

Tabby Tom

4 kittens

?

1 All About Me

18 Clifton Road
Hawsley, Londres
Angleterre
29th December

Dear Marie Cerveau,
 I am writing to you because mon school says you are my Exchange Français and I thought peut être vous might like to know quelque chose about moi and ma famille. I hope you will write and tell me quelque chose about you.
 Ma nom is Susie. J'ai nearly 16 ans et my birthday est January 14th. Mes eyes sont grey/brown et ma hair est long et aussi brownish and une terrible mess. Je n'aime pas school much because je think the teachers sont boring but je ne suis pas mal at biology and pas assez good at French.

I habite in a maison in London. It is ne pas very jolie. But I love it and it has un bon garden. Ma famille est mon père, ma mère, mon older frère et ma older sister et sa chat—Bovril. But now she is ma chat because Sally never gives her un repas. J'aime ma chat beaucoup. Je have done a plan of my family which I am sending with this letter so vous can understand my family better.

In my maison there are:

First mon frère Pete who is très clever and un grand pain in the neck. He is 17 ans et un 'groff', and toujour gets le 'A's in his examinations. He has un place a Nottingham University to do medicin. He is un étudiant de 'driving' but is très mal at that. He is aussi un 'Health Freak' and pense toujours of his body and writes about it dans son diary. I think qu'il est un hypochondriac. Do you have these in France too? Il aime the alcohol but mum ne knows pas. He is also always trying to get off with les girls but is not very bon at it. He used to have une girl-friend qui s'appelle Cilla though now she is, how do you say? passant? He has un très joli ami who is called Sam, whom all the girls aiment beaucoup et me also, but he just thinks of me as Pete's petite sister. Aussi Pete teases me all the time and calls me 'stupide', though I am not, but I get my own back about his glasses. He takes them off when he veut to be a bit more sexy. When you are here, prenez le care when he takes his glasses off!

Ma sister Sally a 21 years. She is très difficile et un rebel. Mum worries about elle all the time and shouts. She habite with her latest boy-friend who nobody here aimes much. Elle est très, très, très pretty and I wish I looked like her. She goes to many parties and spends tout her time at le pub where she works. She used to be a chevaux or should it be cheveux (anyhow a hair) dresser. Je ne sais pas which.

Mon père has a gros stomach and is almost bald. He is gentil but his travail is not very gentil. He is a 'Killer de Pestes'. He has quelque chose which he calls a moustache. Il s'appelle Tony et il smokes cigarettes and pretends il doesn't.

Next is ma mère. She is très bossy and interfering but I think you will really aime her because she is très jolie and funny. Elle mange too much and aime beaucoup le chocolat. Elle s'appelle Jane et elle est a bit grosse everywhere but pretends she isn't. I worry about getting grosse like her. She always wants to know quelque choses about what I am doing and where I am going and avec who.

Sometimes she has the same colour hair as moi but it's curly.

Mes amies are Kate, Emma, Sita, Sheila and sometimes Mary, but my plus close friend who really understands me is Bovril—ma chat—who also aime les boys très much and is always avec them and having kittens.

J'aime les sports, comme swimming and running, and je suis in the school team, but also j'ai hayfever. I hate ma face as it keeps getting les spots and I have to cover it with le make-up which we can't wear at school.

I hope you like my French—please write about yourself and what 'group' you like beaucoup. Do you keep a diary? Je keep a très special book into which I stick everything.

Your exchange amie,

Susie

P.S. Je n'aime pas meat and when I come and stay with you can I just mange vegetables please? Je pense that it is cruel and horrid to kill animals.

P.P.S. Joke:
Question: Why does mon frère Pete, who trouve his body si intéressant, wear his underpants in the shower?
Answer: Because il n'aime pas regarder the unemployed.

2 Organizing Boys, Sex and Work

1st January

I love brand-new diaries. All clean and delicious. Waiting to be written on.

Pete thinks I'm being a copycat, still keeping a diary when his is so famous. He's been a real wally since Cilla went off with David. Anyhow Pete's not the only person in the world keeping a diary. Unlike him, I'm going to write everything that I can think of down, exactly as it happens. If I write something wrong then it'll be like telling lies to myself. That's why I hope this one'll be secret.

2nd January

Only twelve days to my birthday. Can't wait till I'm 16 when I'll be able to:

* get married with the consent of Mum or Dad (Pete would be delighted to get rid of me).
* leave school and get a full-time job.
* leave home with the consent of Mum or Dad (Bovril would have to come too).
* choose my own doctor and decide on my own medical treatment.
* have my own driving licence for moped or motorcycle (not that Mum would let me).
* buy cigarettes (at least now it's legal).
* have sexual intercourse (mmmmmmh).
* get an abortion without Mum or Dad's consent.
* buy premium bonds (already got some from Aunt Jo).
* drink alcohol in a hotel, but only if I'm having a meal (no drinking with Sal down the pub yet).

but I still must have Mum or Dad with me if I'm interviewed by the police (hope this never happens!).

I've got to wait till I'm 17 before I can:

* gamble or go into a betting shop, but I can't make a bet till I'm 18.
* join the armed forces, though Mum and Dad still have to approve.
* get a regular driving licence for cars but not for heavy lorries.
* go to prison.

But I'm jealous that Pete, this year, when he's 18, can:

* see an '18' film.
* get a cheque book and credit card.
* vote (maybe when I can vote I'll help change the government).
* apply for a mortgage.
* buy alcohol in a pub and drink it there.
* give blood (yugh).
* leave home, live with whoever he wants to, and get married without consent (won't be to Cilla, that's for sure).
* change his name without Mum and Dad's consent.
* see his birth certificate, even if he's adopted.
* be a member of a jury.
* get his own passport without Mum or Dad's signature.

3rd January

Pete's sex mad. Seems to be already thinking of trying to put his 'medical knowledge' into practice. He's got a book out of the library about human behaviour. It has a bit about why people are attracted to one another. I'm sure it's all just about sex, but he says it's 'useful stuff' knowing how people choose mates. Says it all happens by 'sexual sequencing'. When you meet someone at a party or something, whether you are first attracted to them or not probably just depends on looks and ways of dressing (but Pete says it's probably smells like pheromones, as well). After that a kind of game begins which is stopped if one or the other person doesn't want to go on. Pete said the problem was when one person wanted to go on and the other didn't—like him and Cilla.

His book says the 'courtship game' (sounds like something in ancient history) starts with looking at each other's bodies (the 'looking stage'), then gazing into each other's eyes. Then comes the 'talking stage' when you are finding out about one another; then a bit of touching, not the proper stuff but sort of disguised, helping you off with your coat, or taking your hand to help you across a road. Next, a bit more touching, like your bodies coming into closer contact, brushing against one another as if by accident. Things get to a slightly more intimate stage when you actually hold hands. Then comes the great leap to the kiss, followed by more serious touching and fumbling. Pete said I was too young to hear the next stages as they were classified '18'. Mum says Pete's got a one-track mind and that he ought to go and talk to the family doctor about it. Pete said, 'Hope she's got all afternoon.'

4th January

Can't keep up. Pete's lost Cilla and now fancies Sandy. But Sandy fancies Sam, so Pete's been trying to go out with Brenda, who will go out with anyone. However, Sam's going out with Joanna, so Sandy's going out with Randy Jo, who actually fancies Emma. I fancy Sam, but I'm not going out with anyone. Maybe I'll never find anyone to go out with and I'll die an old maid.

5th January

Not a good way of starting the first weekend of the New Year—
sitting here, fed up with work and not getting *anything* done.

Pete's admitted to me he's tried cannabis! (I'm putting it in my
blackmail book for when he gets difficult.) Said it was last
year—with Cilla. Asked him why it was OK to smoke cannabis but
not cigarettes. He said it wasn't OK *at all*. At the time he'd thought it
was harmless but he'd found out that smoking a few cannabis
cigarettes had the same bad effects on your lungs as smoking more
than twenty normal cigarettes, and it wasn't any better for your
brain. I wouldn't touch them—they screw your life up, and the
people who sell drugs to children should be hung.

6th January

Every time I sit down to start revising for my mock GCSEs, I just
panic. I get this awful sick feeling in my stomach and rush off to the
toilet. Then I make myself another cup of coffee. How does Pete do
it? His room looks and smells like the local council tip, his love life's
a mess, his spots are like lunar craters and ten times worse than

mine, but he *does* have his work organized. I just flit from book to book—from maths to biology, French to history, physics to English lit and lang—getting absolutely nothing done. Seven subjects seems laughable. Mocks in two weeks—should have worked in the Christmas holidays like boring Mum kept on and on to me about. Don't know why it makes me furious, her always being right. Not that I'd let her know.

But anyhow, who works at Christmas? No way I'd miss the parties, plus my friends wanting presents which were 'just right'. Multicoloured boxer shorts from the Sock Shop for guess who (S). Mum and Dad are the worst. It's 'Anything you've made would be lovely.' Why can't they be the same as everybody else and like what I *buy* them? Got Dad a pair of red braces—really with-it. He said they were just what he wanted, then I found them in the Oxfam pile on New Year's Day. (Not sure what a Third World flood victim would make of them—use them for holding up his house?). Got bright scarlet frilly knickers for Mum, to jazz up her sex life—but think Pete's now got them at the bottom of his wardrobe with his porno mags. They're like teenage mags, but everyone has their clothes off.

7th January

Can't concentrate—my mind keeps coming back to everything I should be doing and still can't. I'm a world-class expert in excuses—got to ring my friends to find out what they're doing, got to clean my room (even that's better than working), got to find my blue, crippled 'chewed to nothing' pen. I've got five, but it's the only one that feels right and it's been lost a week. Worst thing is I've fallen out of love with Bovril. She shat on my bed last night—Mum made me clear it up which made me puke.

Think I'll make a list of suitable boys for me to love:

John—8/10—passable, not a bad kisser (once at Christmas), lives three doors away, in my class, a bit juvenile, into Goth, think he dyes his hair, farts a lot—don't think I could live with so much smell.
Sam—10/10—desirable but doesn't seem to know I even exist. Pete's best friend, self-confident but not a poser. His dad's a leader too—a medical scientist—an Immu . . . something.

Ram—7/10—Sita's older brother. Really attractive but a bit shy.
Mark—2/10—the pits. Sixth-former and a nobody boy—I'd rather
go out with his 7-year-old brother.
Andrew—5/10—OK but in my year. Big-headed—tries it on with
all the girls—even me. Smells of fags and wears white socks.
Winston—8/10—very fit and athletic.
Mike—the midget. Nice, friendly but doesn't really score as he
seems to prefer boys.

8th January

Back at school. I never want to look at a French book again.

9th January

Revision. It's no good, it won't go away. Kate's for coasting along
and then slaving for three weeks before exams. Can't doss about
with GCSE though—so much depends on the teacher's opinion.

   Still hiding my last term's report from Mum and Dad. What some
of them say is not brilliant to say the least. Typical Mum asked
where it was. I said the school had decided not to give them out.

REPORT

English

*Not good — though she could be if
she spent more time in class concentrating
on her work and less talking to her
friends. She also has irritating lapses
of attention in class.*

   J. Jensen.

Physics

Oh dear — Susie not only doesn't do her own work properly but she distracts others as well. I have no idea whether she is any good at this subject. Her homework is always late and when it is handed in it has more to do with flights of fancy than with fact. Having catpaw marks all over it doesn't help its legibility.

O. Boil

Biology

Susie could do very well in her GCSE and might even manage an 'A'. However she must continue to work hard, right up to the examinations, to achieve this. She seems to have a particular interest in the workings of the human body. I wish her luck.

N. Smellie

French

Susie has not kept up her interest in this subject. Her efforts to do absolutely nothing have paid off.

G. Slazenger

History

This is a confident, if rather over-gregarious young lady. Her essays, though informative, are rather slapdash. She needs to improve the organization of her study periods and homework. Recent history and discussion are her strong points.

Trekstring

Maths

Susie's performance is difficult to judge, as she has been away for a great many lessons this term. Much work is needed. When she is present, she tends to blow hot and cold, having periods of extreme activity followed by periods of quiet relaxation.

P. Pie.

P.E.

She has great ability but prefers not to use it.

K. Court

Form Teacher's Report

There are certainly some strengths here, and Susie is a most likeable person, BUT... she'll have to try harder. I think it would help if you would come and discuss this report with me please. Susie needs to improve her working methods if she is ever to succeed to the best of her abilities.

M. Rogers.

Head's Report

Patchy and rather disappointing. I feel that Susie really could do better than this. Her behaviour has not always been as good as it might have been either.

I. MacIntosh

I think there must be a special book of clichés for teachers to use in school reports. It probably has translations as well, like:

'could do better if she tried' = 'totally hopeless'
'has great potential' = 'maybe but I've never seen it'
'outstanding work' = 'never turns up with homework'
'contributes well to discussions' = 'never stops talking'
'must beware of complacency' = 'bone idle'
'must apply herself better' = 'applying herself to work rather than flirting with boys might just help'.

Anyhow, I've decided I'm going to get French GCSE, become Prime Minister, and put the education system back together again. Lucky about outside moderators, but I'm not sure how much it will help. Don't know whether schools are for passing exams, for acquiring knowledge, or for keeping teachers off the streets.

10th January

Even writing to smelly old Aunt Pam and embarrassing and prostateless Uncle Bob is better than working. I put:

Dear Aunt Pam and Uncle Bob
It was lovely seeing you at Christmas. Thank you for the lovely present and delicious lunch. The present was just what I wanted. How are you? I hope you are both well. Thank you again . . .

Couldn't think of anything else. Certainly wasn't going to tell them about my non-existent social life. Uncle Bob's been on at me about my boy-friends since I was 6. It only filled three lines. Couldn't even remember if they'd given me tights or a scarf—both day-glow pink which is what confused me. More for the Oxfam pile. There will be a very hot person wearing pink tights, a pink scarf, and red braces. Bet Mum insists I wear them when we next visit. She'll go on about hurting Aunt Pam's 'feelings'. What about my feelings? Being made to look a twit. Don't think Sam, or anyone else, would fancy me if they saw me in those. At least Aunt Jo's better at presents. Money—just what I wanted. Mum thought it was very generous as she is having a bad time in Germany.

11th January

Forgot what the homework was that had to be in tomorrow.
Phoned all my friends. Panic made worse—they'd all already
done it. Kate and Sita had even gone off to the shops. Never
asked me did they? I just can't cope—but Mum said she'd help
sort it out. Anyhow Mary told me that John is going to chuck
Kate. Says she's 'a slag'. He's one to talk.

List of birthday presents I'll leave around for everybody to see.

SUSIE'S BIRTHDAY LIST

Stripy red jumper
Polaroid camera
Blue dress in window of Top Shop
Leather jacket
New bike
Money
Music centre (there's a cheap one
on special offer in Boots
New brain
Return ticket to Australia
(or even one-way with GCSEs
coming up)

12th January

Pete's in a sulk. Bawled me out for using the rest of his acne cream. Says he needs it more than me. Told him that men with pits on their face are great—like Bryan Adams. Noticed Pete had this great graze on his cheek between the spots. He was furious I'd noticed. Sam and him had been riding Sam's new motorbike and had skidded on a bend. Luckily they'd been wearing cràsh helmets and the bike was only slightly bent. Pete said he'd kill me if I said anything to Mum or Dad. More blackmail material for the future.

13th January

Mrs Smith, who lives two doors away, is giving me some tips on how to sort out my work. Turns out she used to be a teacher. This week we're concentrating on:

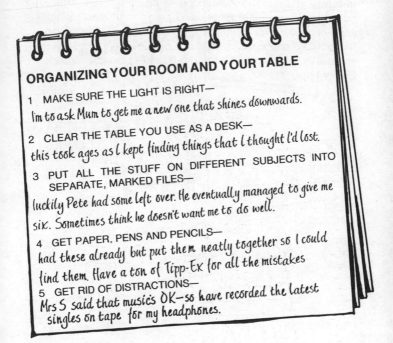

ORGANIZING YOUR ROOM AND YOUR TABLE

1 MAKE SURE THE LIGHT IS RIGHT—
I'm to ask Mum to get me a new one that shines downwards.

2 CLEAR THE TABLE YOU USE AS A DESK—
this took ages as I kept finding things that I thought I'd lost.

3 PUT ALL THE STUFF ON DIFFERENT SUBJECTS INTO SEPARATE, MARKED FILES—
luckily Pete had some left over. He eventually managed to give me six. Sometimes think he doesn't want me to do well.

4 GET PAPER. PENS AND PENCILS—
had these already but put them neatly together so I could find them. Have a ton of Tipp-Ex for all the mistakes

5 GET RID OF DISTRACTIONS—
Mrs S said that music's OK—so have recorded the latest singles on tape for my headphones.

It's unbelievable—Mark (he only gets 1/10 now) is going out with a third-year—baby snatching. She's not only ugly with no sign of tits but is stupid as well. He's got no taste, which is why I don't fancy him. One thing about having a birthday and growing up—it makes you feel really embarrassed looking back at when you were 13 or 14. Especially reading my old diaries. I can't believe the things I wrote. Absolutely cringe at what I wore, who I fancied, and who was my idol. Started to think, ugh—will I look back when I'm 18 or 19 and be horrified about what I am like now?

3 Sweet Sixteen and
Never . . .

14th January

MY BIRTHDAY!

MY BIRTHDAY!!

MY BIRTHDAY!!!

MY BIRTHDAY!!!!

Nice not being at school on my birthday. Was sure nobody would have remembered. Pete's first words to me were, 'Just because you've reached the age of consent doesn't mean you've got to say yes.' Sam won't remember. He's still going out with Joanna. I pretend I don't mind because I really like her, but it actually makes me totally miserable. Don't think anyone likes me. And nobody remembers Christmas and birthdays if they come together. Mum and Dad could have been a bit more thoughtful when they decided to make me.

Most of the time Mum's a real piss artist—fuss, fuss, fuss—but sometimes she's wonderful. Gave me a 'surprise' tea party. Kate, Sita and Emma all came round. Why couldn't Pete have invited S? He invited Randy Jo instead. Even Sally came, skived off work. I'm sure she'll get the sack. Miss her not being at home.

MY PRESENTS:

Mum . . . knickers, M & S stripy jersey (as originally modelled by Mary Poppins—according to Pete) and a James Dean poster—dishy.

Dad . . . a second-hand bike to replace the one stolen last month. (Wasn't surprised as I've been riding his. Would have loved a new one though—this one just means more punctures to mend.) Also gave me a crash helmet, which I *don't* want.

Pete . . . forgot (he owes me for eight birthdays and six Christmases).

Sally . . . ear muffs, make-up paint box, and invite to the pub. Still no official alcohol though (don't think Mum approved).

Kate . . . Percy Sledge tape she'd recorded herself. Think she likes it more than me.

Emma . . . chocolates and two little cat brooches. Sweet.
Sita . . . a really pretty silk scarf.
Randy Jo . . . forgot (though suspect it was him who donated a couple of gas releases during tea).
Bovril . . . think she's been at it again—so it'll have to be kittens.

16th January

Letter from Charlotte who used to be in my class at school—one of our group. We competed against one another in running—till her dad got a job in Birmingham.

My reply!

> *The cheek of it—your letter arrived dated the 14th, I repeat the 14th. What happens on this wondrous day? Yep, it is National Holiday to the world, in other words Susie's birthday. So I open your letter expecting . . . a pop-up box of chocolates? a cheque for a million pounds? or even (sigh) a little birthday card? What do I find? A measly old bumbly letter with NO happy birthday messages. No presents. No wishes—just absolutely nothing but news of YOU and how much happier you are up there now that your dad's got a job! Enough complaining. Actually I loved getting it, and I LOVE getting letters, even if I can't read your writing. I don't suppose it's my fault I'm dyslexic, or your fault you're dysgraphic—just our parents' and our schools'.*
> *Love . . . your very grown-up friend . . . Susie.*

17th January

Pete's pathetic—a tiny cold and he thinks he's dying. Winge, winge, winge. But as soon as Mum told him there was a letter for him, he leapt out of bed and rushed downstairs. Letter was from the library—five books overdue by a month. I nearly fell downstairs laughing. Pete says I'm basically an unsympathetic person and that I never believe him when he says he's ill; and if I want any sympathy when I get ill, I'd better not expect it from *him*. Told him everybody gets colds and nobody knows anything about them. Nobody but Dr Pete Payne, BMKA (Bloody Medical Know All), that is. Even if he had yesterday off, he hadn't wasted his time. He's written an article for the school newspaper where he's doing a weekly column on health. This week—his own problem—colds. Next week it's hayfever, then skin problems, asthma, headaches, contraception, throwing-up and the runs. He's asked me to write the one on contraception as he thought I ought to learn about it now I'm 16. He gave me his 'Colds' piece to read as an example of the kind of thing he wanted.

COLDS, COUGHS AND VITAMIN C

On average you get between one and five colds a year. These are caused by viruses called Rhino viruses (Rhino meaning nose or nostril, like Rhinoceroses which are named after their big horn.) There are over 100 different types of Rhino viruses and your body's defences are not particularly good at producing antibodies to these viruses, so you can get colds again and again and again.

Scientists have set up a 'Cold Research' laboratory where people are paid to go for their holidays. But don't all rush at the same time because you have to do some pretty weird things there. Some volunteers, who had colds, had to wear three-foot cardboard collars and splints on their arms to stop them being able to touch their nose or mouth. They spent a whole day playing cards with others who didn't have colds. This experiment showed that colds *are* infectious, as the people who didn't have colds caught them. The viruses spread more in the air via coughing and sneezing (the air from your sneeze can get blown out of your nose at over 160 kilometres an hour) than on your fingers after picking your nose. (You still shouldn't do that, or only when friends can't see. I think it's a disgusting habit—especially eating it afterwards, even if it does taste good.)

On the other hand *[Pete's got first booking for the repeat of this experiment]*, a group of nine people with colds spent one and a half minutes each kissing someone without a cold. Surprisingly, only one of the kissed group caught a cold. (No, they don't think you can get AIDS by kissing either.)

So why do all you horrible people get snotty and drippy when you have a cold? Well, there are tiny gland cells in your nose, and these make small amounts of sticky fluid which, along with your nose hairs (yes, you all have them), act as trappers of dust and other nasty things, and stop this gunge from getting into your lungs. When the viruses invade your nose, the cells and glands swell up, feel sore and produce more snot.

So does being 'cold' make you more likely to get the virus? Most people think so, but they're probably wrong. To find out, they got people to stand in buckets of cold water, and even to take long cold baths. None of these things made them more likely to get colds.

Linus Paulin, who won a Nobel prize for peace and another for chemistry, said that taking Vitamin C stopped you from getting colds. This has been tried by many people but so far experiments haven't proved that it works.

Antibiotics are no good for colds. They're only good at killing bacteria, not viruses; and it's viruses, not bacteria, which cause colds. Common sense (that's what I hope we've all got in common) should tell you the best way of preventing colds is sneezing into paper handkerchiefs and then throwing them away. (No—preferably not your snot rag which your girl-friend is going to cry into.) If you do get a cold, you'll have to live with it till it goes away.

Millions and millions of pounds are being made by drug companies selling 'cold cures' none of which cure colds, though some might make you feel a bit better. You'd save money by just buying good old paracetamol (so my friendly family doctor tells me), taking hot drinks and trying to get somebody to give you some sympathy (definitely not my sister).

I'll never forgive him—telling the whole school. I threw his mug of last week's coffee at him that he'd been growing new and disgusting strains of fungal penicillin on—and yelled that it was him who said it wouldn't make any difference to his cold—getting soaking wet and having antibiotics. Dad was furious, because it did make a difference to the carpet.

Anyhow, I was interested in what he said about Vitamin C. We'd just done that in school and I thought it cured something called 'scurvy' when your gums bleed and your teeth all drop out. Mrs Smellie said they'd done an experiment on sailors with scurvy in the eighteenth century and had tried giving different groups of sailors cider, sulphuric acid, vinegar, sea water, mustard, two oranges and two lemons, and a ship's normal diet. We were being taught about 'controls', and the question was whether this was a controlled experiment. I said no—but Pete said that I'd got it wrong—the *ship's diet* was the 'control'. He explained that without having one group of sailors who didn't have anything extra they wouldn't have been able to tell whether the sailors had just got better with time alone. Anyhow, this experiment showed that the sailors who had the oranges and lemons got better and the sailors who had the other things or nothing didn't. It wasn't until a hundred years later they knew it was Vitamin C in the oranges and lemons that had done it. Maybe Linus Paulin will be found to be right in another hundred years.

18th January

Mocks have started—no comment.

19th January

Mum has had a nightmare that the librarians from the local library are out to kill her. She dreamt they were stationed with guns at every window and door of the house, with no escape. They were chanting 'bring back the books, bring back the books' and 'pay your fines, pay your fines'. No more driving lessons till Pete takes his books back. Mum thinks it's really mean on the other people wanting the books. Pete said he'd return the books but dream interpretation was rubbish. He'd had a dream about being chased while naked and riding a burning horse down a long corridor full of people.

Makes me almost believe that dreams are kinds of messages—I'm sometimes dreaming about a fire engine when I'm woken up by my alarm bell. No one seems to know whether dreams are just a waste disposal machine for unwanted thoughts, or whether they are DEEPLY meaningful. One of

Pete's unreturned books was on the interpretation of dreams. It fell open at the appropriate page so he must have been reading it.

Being chased—dreamers want to escape from someone. The person chasing them can also represent some aspect of the dreamer that they are unhappy with.

Riding—a fairly obvious sexual symbol, though there is commonly fear as well as desire.

Nakedness—depending on circumstances, and on whether the dreamers are embarrassed and the crowd takes any notice, this can mean inferiority, inadequacy or, alternatively, a desire to be different.

Fire—means passion and danger, and often that thoughts about sex are causing trouble.

Corridor—a feeling that you want to return to your mother's womb and security.

If this is all true Pete's got problems, but it seems to me that you can interpret dreams any way you want to, like the stars.

23rd January

Louise was doing art though now maybe she's not. She's having second thoughts as she was crucified by Mrs Saicops, her art teacher. Sometimes teachers can be really cruel. She said that some pupils have application and no talent but they'll probably do all right, but that Louise has neither application nor talent. I think this is shitty and not even true. It's straight-up bitchiness because Mrs Saicops doesn't like Louise. No knowledge of psychology these teachers. If *I'm* told I'm bad at something, it makes me mad, and I become bad at it so as to fit in with what the teachers think. Louise was so upset she was crying.

4 My Writes and Animal Rights

27th January

Louise's dad had it out with Mrs Saicops about art. Glad it wasn't my dad. I'd be acutely embarrassed—but it worked. Mrs Saicops praised her last life drawing—creep.

Dad can't understand my new maths. Nor can I. He kept asking me questions, just as all Pete's friends were arriving to watch the big match. Mark and Sam came with Randy Jo. Dad talked but I didn't listen, and he left in a peck. I changed into my new stripy jumper and 501s. It's a bit too clingy, so I changed out again. Can't see myself wearing it in public—despite Mum nagging I never wear it. Football's boring—I don't know who anyone is. Wrongly thought I was supporting Sam's team. Made some remarks about Joanna—weren't all nice, weren't all nasty.

One advantage of older brothers—they do have friends.

29th January

Finished mocks—still no comment!

3rd February

Note from Mrs Smith about keeping up with my work plans.
Want to watch telly—great programme about snakes mating.
Have to miss it though—got to work.

ORGANIZING YOUR SUBJECTS

1 Write a list of all the subjects you are doing.

2 List them from the ones that you know least about to the ones you know best.

3 Then list for each subject all the bits of that subject you should know.

4 Keep each subject in its folder to stop them from getting muddled up.

Afraid in my list everything should be top. I'm stopping myself panicking, so here goes:

FRENCH ('orrible)
BIOLOGY (so many facts to learn)
PHYSICS (great but difficult and awful teacher)
MATHS (no comment)
ENGLISH (sort of OK)
ENGLISH LIT (OK)
HISTORY (more OK)

Fed up with work, there must be more to life than this. But Mrs Smith says 'the more you can do today, the less you need to do tomorrow'—and working will make me feel less anxious.

Can't find my French book—not that I really looked. My biology list looks like this:

Life Classifications, Bacteria and Viruses, Fungi, Foods and Feeding.

Green Plant Nutrition, Animal Nutrition, Water Uptake, Blood and Lymphatic System, Respiration, Excretion.

Temperature Regulation, Sensitivity, Co-ordination and Response, Support and Locomotion. Reproduction: Plants and Humans, Genes, Evolution, Ecology.

Doesn't seem so bad written out like this. Eighteen topics, say two hours for each. This almost seems possible.

4th February

Want a Valentine's Day party. No chance of Mum saying yes—not after Sally's breaking-up party five years ago! How does Mum do it? She always knows when I'm lying, like my 'non-existent' school report. She asked me whether Kate and me had been smoking in my room. I said, 'Of course not, Mum. Why do you always pick on me? You know I'd never smoke.' On and on. 'Don't lie to me—I know you have, haven't you?' 'No, honestly Mum, it wasn't me.' Must be the way I answer, or perhaps it's the smell. She's like an awful firework—we'd just lit up and—bang—she appears out of nowhere.

I'm sure I'll die of boredom before lung cancer gets me. The same old lecture. I know it's wrong—she doesn't have to tell me. And it doesn't help, her telling me again and again that 'The number of people dying from the effects of smoking is the equivalent of a jumbo jet crashing every day. That it's not just lung cancer that it causes, but heart disease and bronchitis. That once you've started, it's much more difficult to stop.' I'm not interested in what's going to happen to me when I'm an old hag in fifty years' time. Anyhow I don't smoke very often, and I'm not going to get addicted, and I wouldn't dream of smoking if I was pregnant. No way I'd want to harm my baby. (Not that I'm going to GET pregnant for ages.)

5th February

Pete wants Bov to be in an animal experiment. He saw this TV programme about a link between two parts of the brain that gives us our sex drive. Seeing Bov at it all the time, he said she'd be ideal to experiment on and for him to look inside her brain. But there might not be anything in there, even if her tummy is full of kittens.

I think it's cruel to do animal experiments, particularly on Bov—after all, she must have feelings. Discussed it with Bov who wasn't much help. I joined an 'Anti Experiments on Animals' group in the 'Animal Rights' phase of my life when I was 14. They said there was no point in testing drugs on animals because humans are different from animals, and some drugs tested on animals have been shown to be not safe for humans. As for using animals for making and testing cosmetics—just so you can look beautiful. Nothing will make me beautiful anyhow.

It's so annoying arguing with Pete. I know some of my arguments are correct but the words just don't come out right.

He says I only give a bit of the argument. There have been experiments on animals to do with drugs that are saving *lots* of lives. Animal experiments were essential in the development of the vaccine which meant there was no more smallpox in the world. Also of penicillin, and insulin (the medicine used by people with diabetes), and the drugs used to cure childhood leukaemia. He had lots more examples, but I didn't want to hear them. He had persuaded me that if the experiments are carefully done so as to cause as little suffering as possible—then it's OK. We both agreed that setting fire to people's houses because they were involved in animal experiments was *mental* and it's plain disgusting for girls to plaster their faces with animals. It doesn't even look nice.

At the hairdressers I asked whether the stuff she'd put on my hair had been tested on an animal. She said she'd shampooed her cat with it and it seemed OK. Wasn't quite what I'd meant. Maybe the cat was OK afterwards, but I was a mess. Mum asked why I hadn't bothered to brush my hair today.

8th February

At last—my French Exchange has written. Not that she said much. It was all rather formal. All she said was, 'Thank you for your letter. I'll tell you all about myself when you come to Paris. See you soon, Marie Cerveau.' In French. Managed to translate it with the aid of my dictionary (found in Pete's room). Funny, I used to be really good at translating French when I was in France, two years ago.

At last, a birthday present from Pete—a white rabbit with pink eyes. He was given it by Sam, who was given it by his dad, who rescued it from some experiment. Thought of calling it 'Sam', but settled for 'Pinko'. Mum's furious. Says it's going to be her who has to clean it out and feed it, and look after it when it's sick. Don't actually like it much. Don't fancy its pathetic pink eyes.

9th February

NOBODY, NOBODY noticed my new haircut. So much for £14 and for friends.

Started revising BACTERIA AND VIRUSES. To help me remember, I made lots of little notes and stuck them all over the house, above my bed, in the toilet, on the back of the hall door.

RUBELLA:

1) Also known as German Measles
2) Caused by a virus
3) Harmless to person who catches it
4) Very harmful to baby if you catch it when pregnant
5) Can be prevented by having an immunisation against it
6) All girls should be immunised.

GONORRHOEA:

1) Caused by a bacteria-gonococcus
2) Gives a yellow discharge from the penis or vagina
3) Can make you sterile
4) Easily treated with penicillin
5) Quite common in men and women
6) Condoms reduce the chances of catching it.

Pete stuck up a notice saying, 'If you think you've got a sexually transmitted disease your local special clinic number is . . . . . .' Mum went spare—notes about French verbs all over the house is one thing, notes about sexually transmitted diseases is another. Wasn't having her house turned into a public toilet, 'Thank you very much.' Can't understand it—it's only my revision.

Pete's in Mum's bad books anyway. He missed a driving lesson last night—last one before his test. I made things better by telling Mum how many people had probably survived as a result. Pete's not amused. He thinks I'm joking, but while he's learning, I'm on the most efficient but dangerous form of transport known—my bike. I remember when Pete had his accident a couple of years ago. He had a long lecture from the doctor about how 300 people a year get killed and 30,000 injured on bikes each year, and saying that cycle and motorcycle accidents are the commonest cause of death in young people. He's never worn a crash helmet since, and neither have I, but we both know we should. I'd look such a wally with Dad's white blob of a birthday present on my head. I think it's stupid that there's not a law about it. Then I'd have to, and so would everyone else, and we'd all look wallies and I wouldn't stand out.

10th February

Got my own passport from the Post Office today. Ghastly photo—makes me look like Dad. Now I know I'm not adopted. What a way to find out.

⑤ Broken Hearts and Broken Families

12th February

Pete failed his driving test today. This damaged his ego, specially as Sam's passed his.

We're about to have a German invasion. Uncle Geoff, who's married to Aunt Jo (Mum's sister who doesn't smell), has gone off with 'another woman'. Aunt Jo can't stand being by herself any longer, so she's coming over for a bit of sympathy from Mum. Can't see why anyone would go off with an alcoholic, curly headed, midget British Army tank driver like Uncle Geoff. Would have to be even more desperate than me—though Pete thinks that even I won't have any trouble. There are 3 per cent more boys than girls around nowadays, and by the year 2025 there will be 105 men to every 100 women. If Dad left Mum for another woman Pete said he'd go to the trouble of doing him over.

It's scummy—I have to share my bedroom with my cousin Daisy. I know I don't particularly like the name 'Susie'—but Daisy! Daisy was a 9-year-old prat the last time I saw her. I hated her, and her 5-year-old brother, Paul, who used to wet his bed. Always knew because he never got up in the same colour pyjamas he went to bed in. Mum said his bed-wetting was because his bladder wasn't mature yet. Like the rest of him, I'd say. He'd got better with some kind of alarm thing in his bed that woke him up when he peed. He used to tell Pete how he'd dream about wanting to pee in his sleep, and then he'd wake up and find he'd done it in his bed. Got my own back on Mum about not being able to use the phone. She's on to her sister in Germany every day. One day Uncle Geoff's gone, the next he's back.

Couldn't bear it if Mum and Dad separated. Suppose you never know though. I'm sure that I'll never get divorced—doubt whether I'll even get the chance. If it *did* happen to Mum and Dad, I don't think I would be able to speak about it. Hardest thing would be deciding who to go with. I wouldn't want to hurt either of them and make them think I didn't love them as much. Would be specially bad at celebrations and Christmas and things—having to choose. Some things might be better, like I could get twice as much pocket-money. Also I could be with Dad when I wanted to stay out late and didn't want to be hassled about work, and with Mum when I wanted money for clothes. (Dad still can't see why I can't make do with Sal's old clothes. Can't expect him to know anything about 'fashion' in his old M & S suit bought by Mum.)

Kate's parents divorced when she was 4. She couldn't understand why her father went. She's never really forgiven him for what he did to her mum. It was dreadful. She stayed with her mum living off social security and always short of money. She doesn't think people understand how bad it is for the children—they're just treated like a statistic. One in three marriages end in divorce. It was when she went through a bad patch at school recently that she felt she needed her dad most.

13th February

Don't feel like writing today. Feel SO PISSED OFF.

14th February

VALENTINE'S DAY. NO PARTY, NO CARDS, NO RED ROSES.
(Pete promised me something—at least I expect him to remember,
and he knows that I'm desperate.) My Valentine's Day has been as
romantic as a day's outing to Aunt Pam's.

Pete got three cards and waved them under my nose when I got
home. Asked him where his fatal charm comes from—with his
pebble eyes. Never see it myself. He probably wrote them all
himself. Did my moan bit to Mum about having a party. Think
she's cracking.

15th February

Two Valentine cards! One's definitely from Mum. Can tell from the
innocent smile on her face and the exclamations of 'I wonder who
this can be from?' and (from Dad) 'Who's the secret admirer then?'.
The other one—I hope it's Sam, it must be Sam, let it be Sam. Sam,
Sam, is it you?

16th February

It was Sam—Pete made him do it. Totally embarrassed.

19th February

A week off school.

20th February

Daisy and her brother Paul arrive tomorrow—ugh. What a way to spend half-term. Lecture from Mum about being 'nice to poor Daisy'. Lecture from Pete about girls being stupider than boys because more of them are smoking nowadays.

21st February

Am writing this sitting on the toilet. Nowhere else is private. Daisy doesn't seem very upset to me. Just interested in commenting on everything in my room.

22nd February

Daisy's a pain. Must be awful for her, but it's hard always being nice to someone you don't like. She hasn't improved with the years. Aunt Jo's really nice. She's in Sal's old room. Pity it's so small. Daisy and the thing called her brother must have their father's PPP (Pissing, Poor, Protoplasmic) genes. My biology revision has not been in vain. I also got an A minus for my test on bacteria. Paul's sleeping in Pete's room. Pete is none too pleased, especially as Paul wet the bed last night. Just got up and turned the mattress over to try and hide it. Didn't hide the smell.

Got it from Mum that Paul's bed-wetting had started again when Uncle Geoff left. This didn't impress Pete who said he'd go to Sam's if it went on. I offered to go instead. Pete said no way would Sam be interested in MY body. Mum said she hoped that there's no way Sam would be interested in his. Pete was not amused. Seems to have lost his sense of humour. Maybe he's depressed—Brenda not responding to his charms and not impressed by him failing his driving test. He likes teasing as long as it's not him being teased. When Mum asked him if he wanted anything from Sainsbury's he said, 'Yes—some sanity please.' Bov's the only one who understands how I feel about S. If Mum and Dad separated, I'd take Bov—whoever I went with.

23rd February

It's like old times. Charlotte's down from Birmingham for the day. It's her half-term too. Great to see her and catch up. Bit strange at first though, seeing if we were the same people as before.
Luckily she seemed to get on with Daisy OK. She wanted to know if Daisy missed *her* friends, specially at times like half-term. Daisy said 'yes'—but that it would be difficult telling them about what had happened, even if a lot of their parents were divorced too. They'd moved around a lot because of her dad's job in the army, which made it difficult to keep friends. But Germany, where her dad was stationed now, was just like England—same shops and everything. Everyone spoke English.

Her dad was very strict when he was at home—which wasn't much. Daisy's sure her mum only married her dad because she was pregnant with her. Sometimes she even wonders whether he really is her dad. Now he's gone off with her mum's best friend, Daisy's pleased that she's with her mum. She said her parents had argued all the time and in some ways she was glad her dad had gone, but she's sure her mum misses him. She was really angry with her mum and dad for not telling her or Paul anything of what was going on.

24th February

Daisy keeps a diary too! Found me writing mine—I forgot to lock the door while peeing and writing. Perhaps I'll get a bit of peace when I go off to Paris.

Big mistake! Gave Mum something I found in a magazine Aunt Jo bought about 'Having a Party'. Want to keep the pressure up.

✩* HAVING A PARTY ✩

* Limit the numbers you invite by insisting it's by 'invitation only'. If you can run to it, have invitations printed — even very cheaply; but make them instantly recognizable and difficult to copy.

* Take everything down — pictures, and so on. If something can be broken, it will be. Also allow for the fact that the house WILL BE a total wreck afterwards. Cigarette ends get everywhere, as do the pull fasteners to beer cans, and empty beer cans. Even six months later you may still be finding half bottles of whisky stuffed down the back of the sofa. Leave the whole of the next day for clearing up — not just a few hours in the morning. Try arranging for a few hard workers to stay overnight to clean up, but limit numbers to those who are useful.

* Arrange for a couple of boys to bounce and pay them to drink milk all evening. They can keep away gatecrashers. (Gatecrashers are the worst menace — your friends will at least feel faintly ashamed at smashing everything up — gatecrashers feel nothing.) Get the bouncers to throw drunks out before they puke over everything. As back-up — have a parent or some other adult in the house (but not at the party) to help you if things get out of hand.

* Never, never have any of your parents' drink around in the fridge or anywhere else — it will get stolen. It's too embarrassing to search people for hard liquor on the way in so ask them not to bring it. Get them to stick to wine or beer. Try getting your parents and friends to help out with the costs. Wine is preferred and mixing drinks is disastrous. Never have a 'punch' — people will lace it with everything and you'll need to hire an ambulance as well as bouncers.

* Have lots of food—it helps mop up the alcohol, but most people will probably have eaten beforehand. Have things to eat which don't make too much mess. Always have everything disposable—cups, plates, and so on. Have lots of dustbin bags around.

* If you smell cannabis—get the smokers outside on to neutral ground and only allow them back in after they've stopped smoking (thus at least avoiding YOU getting involved with the law). Try having different things going on in different rooms—music, videos, dancing, snogging. Music matters—so it must be good.

* Remember—as host you may have a difficult time at your own party, but it is a long-term investment. Lots and lots of invitations to other people's parties in exchange for short-term hell.

Mum read it and said, 'I'll think about it . . .' I know 'I'll think about it'. It equals 'No'.

25th February

Pete's turned into a goody-goody. He's just trying to impress— but who cares? He said why didn't I write one of my problem page letters to help Daisy, like I'd written to *Teenage Weekly* about being fat. Daisy and I wrote it together:

Dear Early Times Editor,
I am very depressed and lonely. I thought that my mum and dad were happily married. About a year ago they started arguing and shouting at one another. Dad's gone off with Mum's best friend and I never see him. If Dad can go off I'm afraid that Mum may leave too—and I don't know what will happen to me and my brother. Nobody tells us anything.   Daisy – aged 14.

Back to b . . . . y school tomorrow. But a relief to escape Daisy.

3rd March

Pete's now Macho Hero Number One in Daisy's eyes—she
thinks he's 'WUUUNDERFUL'. The letter that Daisy and I had
written to *Early Times*, and a reply, were published in the
newspaper.

IT may help you to know you're not alone—so try talking to
your friends about it. One in every twenty children aged 5
have parents who have divorced. One in five children
aged 16 have parents who have divorced. Each year the parents
of about 160,000 children get divorced. In spite of this, a huge
study of young people found that they themselves were very
optimistic about marriage, and that twenty-nine out of every
thirty wanted to get married and twenty-four out of every
twenty-five wanted to have children.

One reason for the increase in divorce might be because in
previous centuries people lived much shorter lives and would
usually have been married for only twenty years or less.
Nowadays, with people living to over 70, you may have fifty
years or more of married life. No one would pretend that being
together for all this time is always easy, and most couples will
have some arguments and disagreements from time to time.
Other common reasons for parents splitting up are changes in
the way people feel about themselves, and changes in their
attitudes and in what they mind strongly about. Sometimes
people behave in an unacceptable way (sexually or with
violence) to the other person, or are unable to cope with
children; or they have money problems.

It is very rare for children to want their parents to split up, even
if this means the end of arguments, shouting and general
confusion. Therefore almost all children feel very sad, and
sometimes become bitter and angry with the remaining parent.
As parents are caught up in their own anger and upset feelings,
the children often feel left out and lonely, and in spite of the fact
that it is not their fault at all, may also feel that they are in some
way responsible for the break-up.

Try telling your parents that you need to talk to them about what
is going on and what is going to happen: where you are going to
live, who you are going to live with, what school you are going to
go to, where the absent parent is going to live. What young
children *don't want* is responsibility for making any of the
decisions—like which parent they want to stay with.

One of the best things for separating parents to do is to continue to talk to one another and to their children. They must also realize that their children will continue to love them both, and will want to be reassured of the love of both.

We thought you might like to read about the feelings of some of the other people who have written to us about the same problem.

THE thing I am most upset about is my mum leaving when I was two. I am just going through a bad patch at home and school at the moment and it is at times like these that I need my mum badly. My dad is very good though and I am lucky cos he is good as a dad and a mum. I needed my mum a while back because I started having fits and it upset my dad. I think my dad misses her as well but he doesn't show it. I am worried that when I do get married and have kids they won't have a gran from my side of the family.

....

My real parents split up when I was only three. I was very young and didn't understand. Now I live with an aunt and uncle. My aunt is my father's sister. Not long ago they started fighting really badly and I was afraid they were going to split too. I hate them for what they did to me by bringing me up hating my mum. I don't think people should be allowed to get married until they're sure it's going to work. There should be a probation period so if things don't work out there is no harm done. I also think that if people get a divorce their kids should be allowed to live with one parent or the other. I feel that because of my parents' divorce, if my aunt and uncle divorced I would be the cause of their problems.

....

My parents have already separated. It was hard at first, but I realize that my parents are probably much happier now.

....

About three years ago my parents came very close to separating. The thing that is worst is the violence of it all. There seemed to be such hatred between the two of them. My sisters and I didn't seem to be considered at all. The most horrible thing was going to bed and trying to hide under the quilt and singing to myself so that I couldn't hear all the shouting. All that I wanted to do was to ignore it all and pretend that it wasn't happening. It makes you wonder why they got married in the first place—they seem to have no common interests at all. The problem seems to be a total lack of communication and now this has rubbed off on me and I find it very difficult to talk openly and honestly to people.

My parents have separated, but they are not divorced yet. It doesn't feel that bad, but it's not like I'm glad he's gone. It's quite the opposite. I see him fairly often but he has just moved quite far away because of work. I can't say I miss him because I still see him. After he had gone I found it hard to tell my friends, even though most of my friends' parents are divorced. I think all my friends know now, but most didn't find out from me. Some did—but only the ones I wanted to know.

....

I am now fostered after my parents divorced seven years ago. At a younger age, I was very selfish in my views on whose fault it actually was, and 'why did it have to happen to me?' But realizing that I wasn't the only one in this world whose parents have separated, I got on with my life, treating it like a 'fact of life'. It was neither of my parents' fault. In my mind it was just one of those common factors that neither could live with the other any more. Not meaning that they hate each other but just that they had difficulty putting up with one another. Of course I still cry and wish it hadn't happened, but it's now too late to turn the clock back. As far as I am concerned you just have to get on with life, otherwise you don't get anywhere and become one big dropout!

....

I used to wonder whether I was adopted or something, that maybe Mum and Dad were not my real mum and dad and they had never told me. It's not that I'd mind being adopted. It's just that I'd like to KNOW. I worry about everything, and get myself so worked up I can't sleep. I lie awake until the problem is solved in my mind.

6th March

I don't think the German invasion are going to be with us much longer. Aunt Jo's been found a temporary army house somewhere, until things are sorted out. Just when I've become Paul's heroine. At least one boy likes me, even if it's a bed-wetting 10-year-old. It's because I encouraged him to send off a green crisp he found in a packet of Salt and Vinegar, with an 'it's not good enough' letter. Five packets came back by return of post—one given adoringly to me.

    School meeting about Paris trip today—sounds great.

6 Drunken Louses

14th March

Only just got my diary back. There are some nice people in the world. I was sure someone had stolen it and accused everyone in sight. Pete, Mum and Daisy were the prime suspects because they're all so nosy. I really upset them—it's a wonder I've any friends left. Don't think they realized how unhappy it made me—not having it. I hate losing things. Couldn't think of anything else at first. Was really angry, but then I began to forget about it and decided not to keep another diary. A parcel arrived for me today, couldn't understand it as it wasn't my birthday or anything. Don't know where it came from—no note or anything, just my diary. Hope someone had a good read—as long as they don't know me, that is!

15th March

Paris tomorrow—mell idea. Got to be up by 5.30 a.m. and at school by 6. Dad says he'll take me. My room's a complete tip. Don't think anything I've got suits me. Mum's furious and says I can't go till my room's tidy. No sympathy for the fact that I'll look a complete Sharon—she even likes the way they look!

Pete's promised to look after Pinko while I'm away.

16th March

Fantastic. Kate, Emma, John, Sheila and I all sat on the back seat and shared our lunch. Wished Sheila had sat at the front as she was threatening to throw up all the time. When we got to France, we waved at all the Frenchmen in the cars behind. Good response! Different from back home. Wish Sita had been able to come too, but her parents wouldn't let her.

We stopped off for coffee on our way through Paris. Saw the Eiffel Tower over grey rooftops. Went down the Champs-Elysées past the Arc de Triomphe, over the Seine, dirty like the Thames but with all these beautiful barges with gardens on them, and

children triking round their decks. Wish I could live on one of
them. It's going to be a really good holiday. Coffee, cakes and
wine all the time. Mr Rogers, our form teacher (who used to
teach Pete 'the facts of life' and has been in the school for ever)
is in charge. He refers to me as 'clever Pete Payne's little
sister'—he's another creep but a nice one. He always runs the
French trips. I think either he's having an affair with the French
mistress, Miss Slazenger (who also comes), or he has a French
mistress in Paris!

19th March

Chère Diary—je suis très fed up with this exchange business.
J'arrived here three days ago and je ne peux comprend pas un
mot of what anyone is saying to me. Totally fatiguée by the end
of the day trying to understand and to parler la langue. Madame
Cerveau is very gentille to me. Much better cook than Mum but
she doesn't understand about moi not eating meat. She couldn't
have understood my letter and I can't explain now. Madame
looked très upset when I left her best roast veal. I'm definitely
going to count snails and frogs' legs as meat! Had to give in over
fish or they'd have been convinced I was mad—but I won't tell
Pete. I share a room with Marie—but she goes off and sees her
friends without me. I know Madame tells her to stay with
me—but she jamais does. Last night Madame allowed us to go
out to a disco and Marie abandoned me. NO ONE asked MOI to
dance except a real, grease gun midget with spots the size of
saucers. Luckily Madame had insisted on us being back by 10
o'clock—she's very strict—so the agony was short. They all
laughed and said I was a 'tapisserie'—I found out that meant
'wallflower'. I think I'm going to pleut.

20th March

Now I know why I'm so miserable—my period's started— a
week early and I've forgotten to bring Tampax. Mum had
warned me my period times might get upset by travelling. I've
got terrible cramps and haven't even got the Mefenanic acid
tablets the doctor gave me to use when they get bad. I'd been
having time off school each month before I got them. Perhaps
that explains my maths report! These tablets have made all the

difference to the agonies—much better than aspirin and the other things I've tried.

Went for a 'promenade' to suss out a magasin that might sell Tampax. Didn't like to ask Madame or Marie. How could I? Only just arrived and immédiatement I'm asking for Tampax. Madame doesn't like me wandering around on my own. Wanted to send Marie's younger brother with me. No way. At the local supermarché they were right up on the top shelf. Couldn't just sidle out with them. Had to ask twice in my best French, 'Avez-vous de Tampax si vous plaît?' Whole place—packed with old men—went silent. The shop assistant climbed up muttering, 'De Tampax, de Tampax, toujours de Tampax', pulled out the bottom one, and they all fell on his head along with a load of serviettes sanitaire. Quelle horreur! Très, très embarrassing.

23rd March

Madame took Marie and me to Paris yesterday by train. Wicked—took hours through miles of French suburbia. Loved the metro, loved the Quai d'Orsay, loved the open-air markets, loved the Tuilleries where we sat eating baguette sandwiches and drinking coke (along with the other 200,000,000 daily coke drinkers). Madame bought us une crêpe au chocolat for dessert. Used a pissoir outside the Pompidou Centre which played music while I peed. Five francs for a pee seems un peu cher. Un très exhausting day.

26th March

A letter from Pete! First one he's ever written. Not much of a letter though. Think Mum made him do it. All it was, was a scribbled note on the front of a 'Message to Young People'. Said 'Susie—I'm very worried about you—in France with all that wine—so I'm sending this leaflet to make sure you're not getting alcoholic. Hope you find it useful! Your loving and concerned brother—Pete'.

Personally, I would have liked him to have kept the leaflet for himself and sent me some juicy news about things like, 'How he and Brenda are getting on', 'Has Bovril had her kittens yet?', 'What Sam's up to', and 'Have Daisy and Paul gone yet?'.

How to tell when drinking is becoming a problem

- Do you drink because you have problems?
  To face up to stressful situations?

- Do you drink when you get mad at other people, your friends or parents?

- Do you often prefer to drink alone, rather than with others?

- Are you starting to get low marks? Are you skiving off work?

- Do you avoid being honest with others about your drinking?

- Do you ever get into trouble when you are drinking?

- Do you often get drunk when you drink, even when you do not mean to?

- Do you think you're big to be able to hold your drink?

Alcohol Consumption in Different Countries

Country	Consumption of litres of pure (100%) alcohol per year per person
France	13.9
Portugal	13.1
Spain	11.8
Italy	9.4
Australia	9.2
USA	7.7
UK	7.1
USSR	5.7
Japan	4.4

28th March

Although lots of time—there doesn't seem to be any privacy for writing. Even the toilets in other people's houses aren't the same sanctuary.

30th March

On our way home. Relief to be back with my friends again and to speak English for a change. Kate's family was upset she ate so little. John's family were all alcoholics. He was surprised they didn't have wine coming out of the taps, they drink so much. Mr Rogers was sitting on the seat in front, overhearing us. Breathing out heavily alcoholic and smoke-laden breath, he added that it wasn't just the French who had problems: in 1983 the English spent 13 billion pounds on alcohol, 12 billion on clothes, 11 billion on the National Health Service, 10 billion on state education, and 15 billion on defence.

Bit like smoking. The government are total hypocrites, collecting £200 a second from alcohol taxes and only spending 0.1 new pence per second on advertising its dangers. Really depressing. He said that alcohol drinking was involved in half of all murders, one in five of all child abuse cases, over half of all suicides, and a quarter of road traffic accidents where somebody is killed. I'm sure he knows the facts. He informed us that we didn't need to become alcoholics. With alcohol free wines, beers and ciders, we can still look 'hard' and drink at the same time.

Sheila laughed at my Tampax problems. She'd taken hers with her. She'd tried throwing her used ones into the lav, but they wouldn't flush away. She had to fish them out again, smuggle them through the house in a drippy paper bag, and throw them into the dustbin.

Saw an advert for using condoms as we were leaving Dover: 'Taking a condom on holiday with you won't save your life, using one might'. John said it was a bit late seeing it on the way home, and why were condoms called 'French letters'? Mr Rogers didn't know that, but said there was a legend that the sheath was invented by Dr Condom, doctor to King Charles II. But so much for legends, as he also knew (and I wonder how?) that randy Italians in the sixteenth century were using linen sheaths to stop themselves from getting syphilis. Quite funny really, seeing that everybody is now starting to use them again to avoid getting sexually transmitted diseases. Anyhow, Mr Rogers said that if they bothered to go on teaching Latin in schools nowadays we'd know that the word 'condom' actually comes from the Latin word 'condus' meaning 'a receptacle'. Just like having Pete around—getting all these facts ladled out to us. Thought I'd come on holiday to get away from all that.

There was a funny smell when we were unpacking the cases from the bus. One of the bottles of wine John was smuggling back for his next party had broken. He couldn't believe that wine was so cheap in France. Think he's become addicted while living with his French family. They had two bottles of wine with every meal.

1st April

Slept all day yesterday—exhausted after journey back and by playing with Bov's new kittens (two alive, one dead—what's Pete been up to?). Got up knowing it was April Fools' Day but was fooled all the same. On way to newsagents greedy me saw a pound coin on the pavement outside John's house. Tried picking it up—burst of laughter from behind a hedge. He'd stuck it down with Super Glue. Total failure at catching Pete out. Even tried 'Brenda's on the phone' to get him out of bed, and he's much too clever for the salt in the sugar trick. Did catch Dad with my monster box of chocolates marked 'SUSIE'S CHOCOLATES—DO NOT TOUCH'. A great springing monster bonked him on the nose when he tried stealing one. Think he was more annoyed at getting caught out than anything else.

Pinko's got anorexia. Either that or she's been starved. Pete had done nothing! The cage was filthy and if she did get anything to eat, it was because Mum stuffed an occasional cabbage leaf in. Seem to have got fat in France. I was 62 kilos this morning.

4th April

At last, with her huge experience—ha ha, Louise has started to write her guide to boys . . .

MY GUIDE TO BOYS

by Louise Heathers

BOYS . . . BOYS . . . BOYS . . . BOYS . . . BOYS . . . BOYS
—or why I hate them. When I most want them to notice me they don't. I spend hours getting done up and they don't even notice. I suppose it might bring a bit of excitement into some girls' lives but I just find it obnoxious. When I'm insulted and sulk and I'm waiting for them to apologize they don't, cos they think it's not macho to say sorry.

Occasionally I have these fantasies about the boy of my dreams arriving on my doorstep with a huge bunch of flowers, ready to whisk me away on a huge red motorbike. Some chance!!!

I try to pretend not to be the slightest bit interested. This actually is an awful lot harder than it sounds. When someone I fancy saunters over to borrow my homework, how am I supposed to say 'No' in a calm collected voice when my stomach is break-dancing and my knees are jelly?

Then all I get for my pains is that they go off with my best friend. Boys like that just aren't worth the bother.

This certainly isn't the way I feel about boys. She's even more desperate than I am.

6th April

No boy with a nose would come within a mile of me at the moment as I stink of anti-louse stuff. Paul's leaving present to the family when he, Daisy and Aunt Jo finally left was nits. Aunt Jo admitted it to Mum in one of their endless phone calls. I had thought it was just dandruff when I felt itchy in France. Hope my nits enjoyed their French holiday. Mum found the little beasties.

Dad—the beastie exterminator—was in his element. He said that in a recent survey asking mums whether their children had had head lice in the previous year, one in three said 'Yes'. But worse was to come. If our heads were looked at by a 'beastie hunting' expert, they were FIVE times more likely to find them than our mums. On average, the beasties have been feeding away on our heads for four months before we even know we've got them. Dad was even willing to give us the facts about the louse's sex life: the life of a louse is a mere three weeks; they like everybody's hair but some more than others; they prefer short hair to long, clean hair to dirty (no, that's not a mistake); they seem to spread only directly by head to head contact, they cannot jump, hop, fly or swim, and they can spend time on several heads a day.

What the head louse does when it gets on to your head—between the hairs—is to take a good bite at your skin (up to 200 bites a day per louse). When it bites, its spit irritates your skin and makes you want to scratch. Having bitten and sucked out a little bit of your blood, it then poos. When you scratch, you rub their poo into the bites and the irritation gets worse. The next thing they do (at seven days of age) is start having sex and laying eggs, which they attach to the roots of your hair. A short, but not such a lousy life after all.

To stop this orgy you first have to find the beast, which is the hard part. Mum needed her glasses to find them as they are nearly transparent and a bit smaller than the head of a match; and the eggs on the hair are pinhead sized and flesh coloured. Dad was really mean and cruel. He said that regular combing breaks the legs off the lice. Life is not so easy for a legless louse and they fall off our heads and die. (If animals can feel pain, then why can't lice? What about Lice Rights?)

Mum made the whole family use the smelly anti-louse lotion. Luckily—if used properly—it not only kills the lice but protects you for a bit against getting them again. We had to leave it on over night, couldn't go swimming for two days after we'd used it (that stops it working), and couldn't blow-dry our hair (heat destroys the lotion's chemical properties).

EASTER HOLIDAYS begin today—so don't have to stink out the school.

7th April

Going to have a spending spree. Blow all my saved money. Phoned up Mary to come too. She said she'd love to—amazed she's actually leaving her boy-friend's side to grace me with her presence.

8th April

Caught up on some gossip with Mary yesterday and had a laugh trying on outrageous outfits in Miss Selfridges. So annoying, unless you're thin and leggy, none of the clothes fit or look good. Mary thinks it's stupid to diet and we're all right as we are. She may be—but I feel less certain for myself. Still, why should we try and be like the models in all the adverts? They're all touched up and specially photographed to look thinner than they really are, anyway. Pete says that boys don't really like very thin girls. Says it's girls' minds and personalities, not their bodies, that matter to him. Stop press: Mary saw him at the cinema without his glasses and fumbling with 'all breasts' Brenda. When I suggested it seemed to be *his* mind on Brenda's *body*, he shouted at me to mind my own b. . . .y business.

7 Glands, Fevers and Revision

10th April

Feel awful—hate myself—especially the bit called my throat which is really sore. My tonsils are like two mountains with someone gouging the tops off with needles. If I survive this I promise never to think those thoughts about Sam again. No sympathy from Mum needless to say. She never believes any of us since she found Sally shopping half an hour after she'd claimed she was at death's door with tonsillitis. Pete just did his 'I am the world's number one budding medic' act—told me to shut up and take an aspirin. Bloody know all. He's only got to get a headache and he thinks he's dying.

What a waste of holiday.

11th April

Worse—Sam where are you? Actually anyone who would be nice to me would do.

12th April

Worse, worser, worstest. Pete still doesn't believe I am really ill. He says it's probably just 'Yuppie 'flu' or ME, whatever that is. He won't come close to me though. Don't want him to, but still wish Sam would.

13th April

Worstest of all. It's supposed to be Good Friday, but it's Friday the thirteenth and ghastly. Mum rang the doctor who said most sore throats are due to viruses or bacteria but you usually can't tell which so just to give me paracetamol or aspirin. Big deal. Aspirin for this, aspirin for that. Thousands of years of medical science and that's all they come up with?

Sam called to see Pete today—didn't even come up to see me. I hate him, I hate Pete, I hate the world. I'm going to stay in bed and starve for ever and ever, and then they'll all be sorry.

14th April

Dragged down to the doctors. Much the illest person in the waiting room. The doctor was OK but didn't seem very interested. She made things worse by poking the back of my throat with a stick. Said she'd send it off to see what grows. Yugh—monsters with claws probably. She also took a whole syringeful of blood. I nearly faded away at the end of the needle.

15th April

Dad did his usual Easter egg hunt. Strange, but I still enjoy these rituals. So does Pete, who stole all my eggs and ate them, saying I was too fat already. Tried to get my own back by saying I'd tell Mum about him and Brenda. She's someone Mum wouldn't approve of. He said he wished there *was* something to tell!

Not much fun having Easter and feeling so awful.

20th April

The nurse from the doctor's rang up yesterday to say, 'She's got glandular fever.' So I am ill. Funny thing is, I don't feel so bad now—just floppy and exhausted, like a wet rag. Pete's been making kissing noises at me since he read the 'Glandular Fever' leaflet the nurse gave Mum. (But I haven't kissed properly since Christmas. It was John, who smells awful and wanted to touch me everywhere. Maybe it was him that did this. Perhaps Kate'll get it too.)

GLANDULAR FEVER

(1) WHAT CAUSES IT?

A virus called the Epstein Barr virus (after the men who first described it).

(2) IS IT CATCHING?

Yes—it is an infectious disease and is spread from one person to another. However it's not very infectious and usually you have to be in close contact with a person who has it in order to catch it. That's why it's sometimes called the 'kissing disease', but kissing isn't the only way of getting it. It can also be spread from one person to another like a cold—by breathing in the virus or swallowing it.

(3) WHO GETS IT?

It is very common, and about one in ten children aged 14 and 15 have had it, often without knowing. By the age of 18, over half of them will have had it. Boys and girls get it about equally, and adults can get it too.

(4) HOW DO YOU KNOW THAT YOU HAVE GOT IT?

You usually get a sore throat and swollen glands in your neck. If it's glandular fever, these do not get better as quickly as sore throats and swollen glands normally do. Other glands may also swell up in your groin or under your arms. Sometimes you even get a rash. You'll feel tired, unwell, and will have a headache and a fever.

(5) HOW CAN YOU PROVE THAT YOU HAVE GOT IT?

You have to see your doctor, who can do a blood test. This will usually show whether or not you have glandular fever (or whether you have had it in the past).

(6) HOW LONG WILL IT LAST?

This varies. Some children get it and then get better so quickly that they do not even realize they have had it. For most, it lasts about three weeks.

First week—very sore throat, swollen glands, temperature; you will feel very unwell and like staying in bed.

Second week—fever going down, and you will feel a bit better.

Third week—you will feel much better; fever has gone, but you will still feel very tired, even when doing very little.

(7) CAN IT LAST FOR YEARS?

Usually you get better in a few weeks, but you may still tire very easily for some further weeks, or months, afterwards. For some people the effects last even longer.

(8) IS THERE ANY TREATMENT?

None at the moment—though you may be given an antibiotic by your doctor when you first have a sore throat, before it is realized that you are suffering from glandular fever. This won't do you any harm, but neither will it help cure the glandular fever because antibiotics don't kill viruses (only bacteria).

The only treatment is to take paracetamol regularly (always check the instructions on the bottle or packet to see how much, and how often to take it). This will help bring your fever down, help relieve the pain in your throat, and will generally make you feel a bit better.

(9) SHOULD YOU STAY IN BED AND REST A LOT?

Whether you stay in bed or not depends entirely on how you feel. For the first week or two most children do feel like staying in bed, resting, sleeping, and having drinks and food that are easy to swallow—jellies, soups, ice-creams. Later on you may still feel like resting and sleeping more than usual. Your body, under these circumstances, is usually very good at telling you how much you can do.

(10) WHAT ABOUT PLAYING SPORTS?

It is not a good idea to do sports in the first three weeks of the illness, and you probably won't feel like it. You may even get very tired after mild exercise for weeks or months, so be guided by how you feel.

(11) WILL IT AFFECT YOUR WORK?

During the first weeks of the illness most children find it very difficult to work and concentrate. When you get back to school, it's best to tell your teachers what's been the matter and they will probably be sympathetic. Show them this leaflet if they aren't! Most children find work a problem for some weeks after the illness because of tiredness, depression and lethargy, but it does get better and everyone recovers.

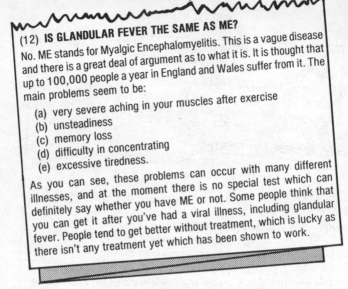

(12) IS GLANDULAR FEVER THE SAME AS ME?

No. ME stands for Myalgic Encephalomyelitis. This is a vague disease and there is a great deal of argument as to what it is. It is thought that up to 100,000 people a year in England and Wales suffer from it. The main problems seem to be:

(a) very severe aching in your muscles after exercise
(b) unsteadiness
(c) memory loss
(d) difficulty in concentrating
(e) excessive tiredness.

As you can see, these problems can occur with many different illnesses, and at the moment there is no special test which can definitely say whether you have ME or not. Some people think that you can get it after you've had a viral illness, including glandular fever. People tend to get better without treatment, which is lucky as there isn't any treatment yet which has been shown to work.

24th April

Kate told me I'd missed a timed essay for GCSE English—will I fail? Made Mum give Pete a note for school. The teachers always think you're just skiving even if you're dying. Bet Pete forgets.

2nd May

Mum spoke to my teacher. Hate her doing that but it seems I haven't missed out on my GCSE. My teacher said that if I had missed an essay, all they would do is take the best of one of the ones I have already done. If it had been worse, and I had missed more, it would've been OK to get a note from my doctor.

Horrible fright today—thought Bovril had broken her leg. She was limping around trying to keep up with her kittens. She's only just back from being 'done' at the vets'. I found this huge great bump and something sticking out of it. She mewed pathetically every time I touched it. I panicked and rang Mum at work. She came home at lunchtime and said it looked like a bee sting. Then I remembered that Bov had been playing around with a bee—trust her to pick the first bee of the year. Felt a real fool dragging Mum back. Especially when she said to leave Bov alone—that it would get better by itself.

Dead bored being around home, dead tired if I try doing anything else. Searched Pete's room—found this book of jokes in his wardrobe (along with three old copies of *Playboy* and a couple of other wank mags). Light relief at last, so cheered up.

If it moves—fondle it.
Don't take the piss out of beer—it needs all the flavour it can get.
Why is virginity like a balloon?—one prick and it's gone.
100,000 lemmings can't be wrong.
Support the wild life—vote for an orgy.
If at first you don't succeed—forget it.
If you've got fluid on the knee—you're not aiming straight.
People who live in glasshouses should have sex in the basement.
Y-fronts prevent fallout.
I'm perfectly well adjusted—but you can fiddle with my knob.
Is Johnny Cash change from a condom machine?
Keep Britain green—have sex with a frog.
Photographers do it in the dark.
Teachers do it with class.
Town planners do it with their eyes shut.
What's brown and taps at the window?—a baby in a microwave.
Rugby players do it with odd-shaped balls.
Adam came first, men always do.
Careful—more than two shakes is masturbation.
Keep pop music live—kill the producer of Top of the Pops.

6th May

Pete's nagging me about the article on contraception. Thinks I've got nothing better to do, just because I'm ill. He's revising away for his 'A's. I should be revising for GCSE, but I can't concentrate. Pete gave me a pile of family planning leaflets, to copy out the best bits. Must be anonymous though—can't have the whole school thinking *I* know anything about it.

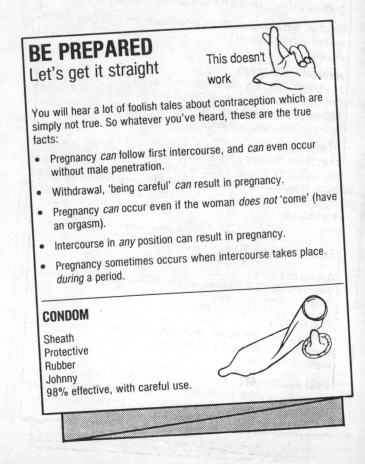

BE PREPARED
Let's get it straight

This doesn't work

You will hear a lot of foolish tales about contraception which are simply not true. So whatever you've heard, these are the true facts:

- Pregnancy *can* follow first intercourse, and *can* even occur without male penetration.

- Withdrawal, 'being careful' *can* result in pregnancy.

- Pregnancy *can* occur even if the woman *does not* 'come' (have an orgasm).

- Intercourse in *any* position can result in pregnancy.

- Pregnancy sometimes occurs when intercourse takes place *during* a period.

CONDOM

Sheath
Protective
Rubber
Johnny
98% effective, with careful use.

HOW IT WORKS
Made of thin rubber and worn over the erect penis, a condom prevents sperm from entering the woman.

MAIN ADVANTAGES
Easy to obtain and use. Man can help take the responsibility for birth control. Can protect both partners against most sexually transmitted diseases and may protect the woman against cancer of the cervix.

Question: What do you call people who use the 'safe period' as a method of contraception?
Answer: Parents!

MAIN DISADVANTAGES
May slip off. Men may find some sensitivity loss during intercourse. Can interrupt lovemaking, although putting condom on can be enjoyed as part of loveplay. Needs care to ensure that no sperm are spilt after ejaculation (coming).

COMMENTS
Must be put on (using a new one each time) before the penis touches any part of the woman's vaginal area, and held in place when the penis is withdrawn. Only use condoms with a British Standards Institution 'Kitemark' on the pack. Freely available from garages, chemists, etc.

THE COMBINED PILL

Oral contraceptive
Over 99% effective, if taken properly.

HOW IT WORKS
Contains two hormones—oestrogen and progestogen. Taken regularly it stops ovulation (the release of a woman's egg each month).

MAIN ADVANTAGES
Easy and convenient to use. Gives regular monthly cycle, often with reduced amount of bleeding, period pain and premenstrual tension.
Does not interfere with lovemaking.

MAIN DISADVANTAGES

Some women have minor side-effects which normally pass in a few months. The pill appears to be a safe method of contraception but it has only been around 25 years and we still may not know some of the long-term problems that it may cause especially if it is taken for many years.

DOES *NOT* PROTECT AGAINST SEXUALLY TRANSMITTED DISEASES.

COMMENTS

Does not work if taken over 12 hours late, or if there is sickness or diarrhoea, when a condom must be used. Some drugs may stop the pill working—a doctor will advise. The pill is prescribed by a doctor. Pill users should try not to smoke.

DIAPHRAGM OR CAP + spermicide

97% effective, with careful use.

HOW IT WORKS

A soft rubber device, put into the vagina before intercourse, to cover the cervix (entrance to the womb), and form a barrier which prevents sperm from meeting the egg. Must be used with a spermicide and left in place for six hours after intercourse.

MAIN ADVANTAGES

The diaphragm/cap and spermicide can be put in at any convenient time before intercourse, so need not interfere with spontaneity. (More than three hours between insertion and intercourse just means using additional spermicide). It may protect against cancer of the cervix.

MAIN DISADVANTAGES

Have to get one from a doctor to make sure the size is right. Need to plan ahead so that diaphragm/spermicide are in place before intercourse. Must check every six months that cap is the right size, or after weight gain or loss of more than three kilograms (seven lbs) as size of the vagina may change.

COMMENTS

A spermicidal cream, jelly, pessary or foam (which inactivates sperm) must be used with the diaphragm.

The basic facts

A woman can become pregnant if, after intercourse, a sperm released when the man 'comes', joins with her egg and the egg then settles in her womb. A man and woman who do not want to have a baby can still enjoy lovemaking if they make sure the egg and sperm never meet, or if the egg is prevented from settling in the womb. There are several ways of doing this, but any method chosen must be used properly. No birth control method will work unless it is used regularly—the one time you take a chance could be the time pregnancy occurs!

Different contraceptive methods suit different people at different ages, so ask the advice of your family doctor or your family planning clinic. If necessary, try out one or more methods until you find the one that suits you and your partner best. You are far more likely to use a method regularly and properly if you feel it is the right one for you.

Remember!

If you feel embarrassed about going to your family doctor you can go to any family planning clinic. It's free (look for phone number in telephone book).

'Morning-after' contraception

If you are unlucky and make a mistake with your contraception, the 'morning after' pill is available. This means taking a special dose of the combined pill. It is available from GPs and family planning clinics. The woman can take it up to 72 hours after intercourse.

If you don't want a child—don't trust to luck. *Use a reliable method of contraception.*

14th May

Back at school and GCSE exams in three weeks. Massive catch-up needed. If I fail my exams I'm not sure what I'll do. I'll probably blame myself for being a lazy cow for the last two years—though it wasn't my fault I was ill.

I'll be a complete failure—a nothing. It's terrible pressure, all these exams, specially as I don't know what I'd say to my friends if they asked me how I'd done and I'd failed. Mum says I can only do my best, but whatever she says I know she'll be sad if I don't do well. (Not even sure that Dad knows I'm taking them.) Wish I could turn the clock back and begin my revision again. I've got Mrs Smith's revision plan to work to:

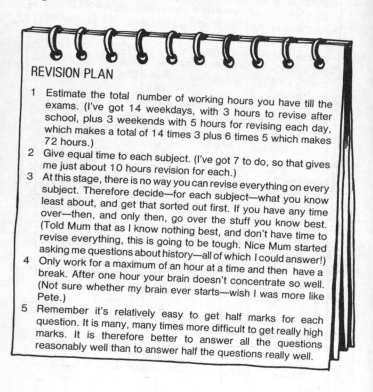

REVISION PLAN

1 Estimate the total number of working hours you have till the exams. (I've got 14 weekdays, with 3 hours to revise after school, plus 3 weekends with 5 hours for revising each day, which makes a total of 14 times 3 plus 6 times 5 which makes 72 hours.)

2 Give equal time to each subject. (I've got 7 to do, so that gives me just about 10 hours revision for each.)

3 At this stage, there is no way you can revise everything on every subject. Therefore decide—for each subject—what you know least about, and get that sorted out first. If you have any time over—then, and only then, go over the stuff you know best. (Told Mum that as I know nothing best, and don't have time to revise everything, this is going to be tough. Nice Mum started asking me questions about history—all of which I could answer!)

4 Only work for a maximum of an hour at a time and then have a break. After one hour your brain doesn't concentrate so well. (Not sure whether my brain ever starts—wish I was more like Pete.)

5 Remember it's relatively easy to get half marks for each question. It is many, many times more difficult to get really high marks. It is therefore better to answer all the questions reasonably well than to answer half the questions really well.

18th May

Revision going well but no time to write diary. Feeling less tired thank goodness. Mum's in a peck about Brenda. Thinks she's a bad influence on Pete. She smokes and goes to pubs, and Mum's sure she's on drugs. (I know she is, and so does Pete!) Bov's in a peck about her kittens being given away. Better than drowning them, but she doesn't understand that.

	MONDAY	TUESDAY	WEDNESDAY	THURSDAY	FRIDAY	SATURDAY	SUNDAY
9.00 10.00							
11.00							
12.00							
1.00							
2.00							
3.00							
4.00							
5.00							
6.00							
7.00							
8.00							

8 Exams and Abuse

4th June

Panic, panic, panic. I can't sleep, I can't stop eating, I can't concentrate. I'm tired all the time, I've forgotten everything I've ever learnt, I'm terrified of everything going blank when I see the exam paper, I can't do any revision as it all disappears again.

Being at school's worse—mass hysteria—everybody as scared as I am! I think the staff are really pissed off. Mr MacIntosh—the head—did one of his 'now then children, don't panic' speeches. Quite scary, with his wire specs, white hair and crinkled face. He looks about seven feet tall up on stage.

 It may be too late to revise now. Most of you will experience panic at one time or another when faced with that dreaded moment when you are first given the examination paper. Some of

the things which will happen when you read it are good. More adrenalin will be pumped round your body, your heart will beat faster, and you will become generally more alert. However some of your reactions may be less positive—being unable to concentrate, thinking your mind has gone blank, feeling sure that you know nothing.

So wouldn't it be good if there were a few very simple tricks to help you cope with the bad aspects of panic? Well, there are. They are things that have been learnt by people who have taken many, many examinations. They can help a great deal, but they need a bit of practising.

What really stops the panic is if, instead of rushing in and being convinced you will never finish the exam paper in time, you spend a few minutes getting yourself organized before you start writing. Many marks may be gained as a result of those few minutes planning.

First—and foremost if you feel yourself panicking when you get the exam paper—count slowly to ten before reading it. This will only take ten seconds but will allow your nerves just that tiny bit of time to calm down.

Second—read the instructions carefully as to HOW MANY questions you have to answer. (You will not get one single extra mark for answering more questions than you need to.)

Third—read the instructions again and find out how much time you have for the examination as a whole. Then divide the number of questions you have to answer into the total time, and work out how long you can spend on each question. (5 questions in the 86 minutes left in a 90-minute exam—after the 4 minutes that it has taken you to do the things listed here—means about 17 minutes for each answer.) Spend ONLY that amount of time on each answer.

Fourth—read each question carefully, decide which you want to answer, and quickly write down notes on everything you know about each one BEFORE you start to write the full answer on the one you know best. The reasons for this are very simple:

a) If each question is marked out of the SAME amount—say 20—to get 12 out of 20 is fairly straightforward; to get 14 out of 20 you have to be very good; to get 17 or more out of 20 you would have to know the topic inside out.

b) If you spend half the total exam time answering the question you know best really well, and then only manage two more answers of the five you should have done, then you might get 41 marks (17 for your excellent one and 12 for each of the others). But if you do all five just fairly well (12 marks each) you will get 60—simple really.

Writing short notes at the beginning—on every question you are going to answer while your mind is still fresh—prevents you from panicking about not having anything to say on the ones you know least about. **'**

He ended by wishing us 'All the very best of luck'—nice but a bit pompous. It's easy for him to say that—*he* doesn't have to do the exams.

Pete's into 'A's. We're not allowed to talk about *his* exams. We get screamed at if we ask how they went. Don't know what he's making such a fuss about—he's bound to do well.

Dad and Mum totally fed up today. They're thinking of going to live somewhere else till it's all over.

5th June

Exams start tomorrow. Resolutions:
I won't panic
I will read the questions
I will look and see how much time I have
I will see how many questions I have to answer
I will write short notes first
I will do my best handwriting
I will have all my pens and pencils and my calculator with me.

HELP!

P.S. I must remember to take my hayfever spray regularly.

6th June

The English exam was easy but I messed it up. Didn't see the question on the last page. So much for my resolutions. I had tummy pains all the way through. Curse periods. I think examiners should make allowances.

It really made a difference—Mum and Dad being so relaxed with me about the exams. Kate's mum hassles her every time she wants to go out. Even on a Friday night she goes on about 'but what about your homework? Have you thought about the revision you need to do for the exams?' Right in front of her friends. It's really not on—would make me want to do just the opposite. What do they think? That we want to fail our exams? At least Mum and Dad seem to trust me (most of the time anyway). They remind me to have rests from work, and they bring me cups of coffee. Mum makes a special effort to have meals on time and to give me treats.

8th June

Maths OK. But Sheila wasn't. She walked out sobbing—half-way through. Everybody looked at her as she went. Nobody could understand. She's the brain.

9th June

Thank God for weekends. Kept to my timetable of revision. One hour biology, cup of tea, one hour history, cup of tea and a walk. All was well till I looked at an old GCSE history paper and couldn't answer two of the five questions. I'll never manage. Rang Kate and Emma to come for lunch. Kate said she couldn't make it for lunch, but came afterwards. I don't think she likes eating. It turns out the reason Sheila walked out yesterday was nothing to do with maths!

She'd been depressed for ages because a man had tried to rape her. It all started a year ago when she got a job working part-time in a café belonging to a friend of her dad. It was OK for the first few months, but then the owner insisted on walking her home, even though she lived very near. During the Christmas holidays every time he walked her home he tried to make her hold his hand. She didn't like it but thought he'd had too much to drink or something. She started to dread going there, but didn't want to give it up because of the money.

One night towards the end of January he was walking her home and holding her hand. Then, still holding her hand, he put her hand in his pocket. She suddenly realized that there was a hole in his pocket, because her hand was touching his skin. She tried pulling her hand away. They were still walking towards her house and she couldn't say anything. When they finally got there he let go and she ran in crying.

She felt she couldn't tell her mum who wanted to know what was wrong. Sheila said that she was just tired, and went up to bed and cried herself to sleep. She didn't think that she would ever hear from him again, but the next week, while she was out, he phoned and her mum said she could work that night. While he was walking her home this time, he actually tried to rape her, but she managed to get away.

She couldn't tell anyone, because she felt partly responsible, but she thought about it all the time. She hated that man and wanted to kill him. Since then she has stopped working, but she sits and goes through it again and again, thinking about what she should have done. It hurt her to think about it—really hurt she said. It made her feel so ashamed and humiliated she wanted to scream. Once, when it got particularly bad, she couldn't even kiss her father. She knew that if she did she'd be sick. Sometimes she blamed her mother and her best friend for not noticing that she was unhappy. She'd hinted but they'd never caught on.

The exams were the last straw—but at least now her parents know. She's reading a book called *Too Close Encounters and What to do About Them*.

Luckily I was able to tell my mum about the flasher who pulled out his shrivelled willy in the cathedral when we were on holiday in France. Mat and Sam thought it was funny—but it wasn't for me.

11th June

History today—managed all five questions—hurrah! All that revision was worth while. French in the afternoon—un complet disastre, et je suis miserable maintenant.

Pete thinks that men like Sheila's boss should have their balls cut off. Mum says you can't do that, though they do need some kind of treatment. Still the same message from her. Everyone (including Pete) should know when to say NO—like my friend Jane did when we were 13 and it happened to her. The only time it nearly happened to me was when some girl-friends and I were coming home across the park after a party. Some older boys followed us home, calling us 'slags'. I've never been so scared. I thought they were going to rape us, especially as another girl, who was a bit drunk, was leading them on. Luckily, they went away after about fifteen minutes. Since then I've followed Sal's tips on being careful:

* If possible I stick to well-lit and well-used routes when going to and from school and people's houses.
* I always try and walk with someone I know.
* I never hitch-hike although sometimes I would like to.
* I never play in or hang around in lifts or toilets (too smelly anyhow).
* I only carry the money I need (if I have any!) and don't advertise it in public.
* I try to tell Mum and Dad where I'm going and what time I'll be home (they always ask anyhow).
* If I go to a party, I make sure I know beforehand how I'm going to get home.
* If anyone tried to touch me in a way I didn't like, I'd say NO loudly and firmly, and tell someone about it.
* If I was attacked, I'd scream and run to where there were other people (better to run than to face the attacker).
* If I couldn't run, I'd scream and kick, or knee the attacker in the balls, squeeze his windpipe, try and gouge out his eyes.

I sometimes wonder why men don't try it on with me. Maybe I'm too ugly or too flat-chested (I think Sally has taken all the boob genes in our family). Pete says I don't need self-defence lessons as I scare men off naturally. Maybe if I wait long enough, someone will come along who will love me for my mind.

14th June

Revision programme gone to pot. Fed up with taking exams. Wish they were all over. Thank goodness my hayfever hasn't been bad this year. Maybe the sprays have helped, or maybe there's been no pollen.

19th June

The big day! THEY'RE OVER and there's a party at Mark's house. Mary came round to get ready at 3 p.m. The party wasn't due to start till 8. She looked brill in her outfit. I was really jealous and had serious doubts about my new skirt, but Mary said it looked great. She's a good friend to have sometimes. I tried some new lipstick—sort of dark rose colour—but it was too dark. I mixed it with some of the usual stuff and my lips ended up looking like a chocolate-covered raspberry. Talking about chocolate—I'm going on a 'no chocy' diet. I still weigh 56 kilos!

We got to Mark's just before 8.30 and I immediately wished I'd worn my 50ls. I felt a bit nervous as I couldn't see many of my mates, though some of Pete's were there, including Sam, so Mary and I went over. Mary was all over him like a bitch on heat and I felt insanely jealous. I stormed off to get myself a drink—hotly followed by Sam, who gave me the 'What's up with you?' line. How could I possibly explain? I picked up my drink and rushed off to the loo. When I came out, I came across Randy Jo and big-breasted Brenda heavily into business behind the settee. Not surprised Pete thinks she's a slag. It's amazing she's not pregnant yet, the way she goes at it.

I sat under the stairs for half an hour drowning my sorrows in drink. Don't know why I drink—it's more a depressant than a stimulant, and what's more I feel rotten next day. While I was sitting there, someone I didn't know tried offering me something but wouldn't say what it was. No way I was going to try it. I think it's mental to use drugs like cocaine, heroin, and amphetamines. They should stay illegal to put people off using them. Though cigarettes and alcohol are drugs too—and I do use *them*. I think it is utterly wrong for people to make so much money from trades that are killing people and destroying so many lives.

John came over to see if I was OK, and for some unknown reason (maybe the drink) I told him all about Sam. John decided I needed cheering up so he took me to meet a mate of his—Charlie—after I had checked the state of my mascara in the bog. He seemed a nice enough bloke, witty and not bad looking—the sort of dark-haired, blue-eyed bloke you'd give your last Rollo to. We talked about music, school (he's leaving this term), and how boring the town is getting. We actually had a lot in common and I felt really relaxed talking to him. He didn't put on a macho-bastard image when his friends came up, which was a change. He asked me if I would like to take a walk outside, which made me a bit nervous. Some boys seem to see this as an opportunity to start french kissing which could put a damper on the situation. I didn't want it to start getting heavy. But I felt no pressure from Charlie and he didn't even fumble with my bra. He wrote down his telephone number and I gave him mine, but it will probably be a one-night stand thing which comes over as the kind of stuff dreams are made of. If he doesn't phone it was nice while it lasted, if he does I'll be over the moon.

21st June

He hasn't rung. Stupid of me to think he would. Wonder if I should give him a ring to see if he's lost my number? I'd look a right fool if he hadn't and doesn't want to see me again. Why am I such a flid? Actually, I'm not sure that I do want to see him again. From something Pete said yesterday, I think he may be into the drug scene.

22nd June

Pact at school between Emma, Kate and me not to eat food that's bad for us. We all feel lumpy after all that nervous eating over the exams.

27th June

So far, I've managed not to eat:

chocolate for two days

cake for four days

sugar for five days

cream for a week

I did feel like a whale, but I'm certainly not a minnow yet. Kate's lost 2 kilos—and she was only 45 kilos to start with. She says she wants to become a ballet dancer. If she's not careful, she'll become anorexic.

9 Flab is in the Eye of the Beholder

2nd July

Dieting didn't last long. We've all stopped except Kate. We decided it was stupid, but she's become obsessed. She wouldn't come to Coles for a celebratory 'end of dieting' tea. She made a feeble excuse about meeting her mother, but I'm sure it's her not wanting to eat. According to Mum, Sal went through a not-eating stage for months, when she was doing her 'O's, but it never got very bad. Mum dug out a booklet she'd got for Sally at the time.

ANOREXIA
Jenny's Story

I'm not sure how my anorexia started. All I do remember is wanting to be as thin as a friend of mine. I wasn't fat or anything. Just average size. But for some reason, I desperately wanted to be thinner, like my friend.

At this particular time—I must have been about 12—I became aware that my brother was thinner than me, though I didn't really start dieting properly then. My mother had always been fussy about what my brother and I ate—mainly because of our teeth. We'd never been allowed biscuits or cakes, just the occasional sweet. You see my father was a big fat man, and my mother thought that there was nothing worse than having fat children as well.

It was in my second year at senior school that I decided it was about time I was the same size as my friend. I can't actually ever remember waking up wanting to diet. It was just a very gradual process.

A year later I was seriously underweight and was diagnosed as anorexic. I was given a week to live if I didn't start eating. I had gone through several changes in my eating habits during that year.

I started off having fruit for breakfast, pork pie for lunch, and a small dinner. I took ages to eat each item as I deliberately cut it into tiny pieces, the same way each day. My meals had to be at rigid times, and any later or earlier would be terrible. I can remember distinctly cutting up my pork pie into very small pieces and sucking each tiny particle of meat. Then my breakfast changed to a small piece of melon, and lunch to a scotch egg. (It had to be a very special one, and if I couldn't get it there was trouble.) I started doing lots of exercises too.

When my family and I went on holiday to our usual place in Cornwall, friends we see there every year noticed the difference in me. As well as me being a lot thinner, they felt my character had totally changed. I was very withdrawn and almost like an old woman. I thought it was childish to play beach games so I sunbathed like my mother. I became very dependent on her and didn't want to enjoy myself like everyone else.

When we got home, each day was the same old drag, and once again my eating changed. Lunch became a chicken salad which only I could prepare. Life was hell for everyone and I cramped the whole family's style. Going out for a meal was a waste of time and money, and not just me but no one enjoyed the experience.

Then things got even worse, with no breakfast, a tiny salad with no chicken for lunch (my parents didn't know), and small pieces of cut-up vegetables for dinner.

The season changed and I remember getting really cold now that it was autumn. My parents became very worried. It was now obvious that something was definitely wrong. (I suppose they had realized that for a long time but hadn't wanted to accept the situation.) My mother feared that I might have anorexia, and said that if I wasn't careful I'd have to be fed by a drip into one of my veins. I got angry with her and told her not to be stupid. How could a person as fat as me be told to eat and put on weight? The fact that I was many kilos less than all my friends never made it click that perhaps I was actually very thin. I continued my regular exercises and went on refusing to eat. I suppose you could say I'd become trapped in a vicious circle and my anorexia had completely taken me over.

However, on 12th November I had to go into hospital. (I was 14 at the time and 163 cms. tall.) I weighed only 34 kilos, but I didn't want to go there at all. I didn't want any kind of help, though I do remember being made to have a small beefburger at McDonalds a few days before and thoroughly enjoying it. I hadn't had one for ages, and had forgotten how nice they tasted. However, there was no way that I was going to admit to liking it. My parents would have given me one more often and eating would have made me feel guilty.

When I arrived at hospital I was told that if I didn't put on 9 kilos by Christmas then I couldn't go home to spend Christmas with my family. Christmas meant a lot to me, and always had done, but my anorexia was so strong I didn't care whether I went home for Christmas or not. I just didn't want to put on weight. In the end I did go home—for Christmas Day only—as I had been successfully forced to eat.

In hospital I had to eat three big meals a day and three snacks with milky drinks containing a high-calorie powder. Each meal took me two hours and each snack took an hour. After each one I had to lie on my bed for half an hour. This was the most stressful thing to have to do. I would much rather have run a mile but there was a nurse supervising me all the time. Everyone was very caring, of course. Every day I got a letter from my mother together with numerous other letters from friends. Eventually I reached my target weight and on 1st February was allowed home. I was relieved to be home again but my treatment continued, and I had regular family therapy meetings at the hospital as an outpatient, either with my family or on my own.

The one thing I can think of which helped me while in hospital was the love and care of all my family and friends. This wasn't the case at first. When I was diagnosed as having anorexia there were lots of different reactions from everyone. My family were shocked and upset. It was difficult for them to understand my eating problems, especially my brother who loves his food. What a lot of people find difficult to understand is that anorexics absolutely love food. They love it so much that they're scared that if they start to eat they won't be able to stop. But their anorexics' powers are so strong that they won't let themselves eat and enjoy food.

My grandparents found it tormenting too. They had never heard of the illness. They thought it had not existed in their day. They found it so weird that I should want not to eat all the time. Even now I don't think they fully understand.

The only person in my family who is anywhere near understanding is my mother. She has had a mild obsession with food so it is easier for her to help me than most other people. It really has been the love and care that she has given me, and the love that everyone else has shown, that has given me the incentive to try and get better—even if I am doing it just for them.

WHAT'S ANOREXIA ALL ABOUT?

Anorexia nervosa is a condition that occurs more commonly than you might think. It's not only girls who have the problem, but it's much more common in girls than boys. One in 200 teenage girls suffers from anorexia but only one in 2,000 boys. It usually starts in your mid-teens (it is much less common before the age of 13). Girls at boarding schools, fashion students, and ballet students are especially at risk.

There are lots of theories as to why it happens. For instance, it is an expression of depression, a response to stress, an attempt to run away from the conflicts of growing up; it's due to a feeling of being totally hopeless at everything; it's a fear of losing control over eating and becoming fat.

One common thread that runs through all these explanations is the stresses and strains being faced at this age by both sexes. The typical woman for instance is expected to be slim, beautiful, brainy, warm, loving, capable, kind, tough, business-like, etc., etc. Ideals that a girl in her early teens may find rather frightening to live up to! To maintain control over at least one thing in her life—her weight—may therefore become an understandable obsession.

One thing all anorexics have in common is that they all over-estimate in their minds how fat they are. Even though they may be thin and underweight, they *think* of themselves as fat.

WHAT ARE THE FIRST THINGS THAT HAPPEN?

- you lose a lot of weight by deliberately not eating and/or exercising a great deal
- you get obsessed with the idea that you are fat and it's a dreadful thing to be
- if you are a girl, you stop getting your periods.

WHAT OTHER THINGS CAN HAPPEN?

- your arms and legs become as thin as sticks
- your hands and feet become blue and very liable to chilblains
- you may not be able to sleep
- you may not be able to concentrate, though you may think you are being very clever
- you get very sensitive to cold
- your skin becomes dry and hairy over your neck, arms and legs
- your heartbeat rate slows down and down
- you may become increasingly sad and depressed
- you may become a compulsive user of laxatives (tablets which make you shit a lot and stop your food being absorbed, but which can also make you very ill).

YOU SHOULD WORRY THAT SOMEONE IS BECOMING ANOREXIC IF THEY:

- become obsessed with food and cooking for others, but don't eat themselves
- get very thin
- seem restless when meals are being served, won't sit down to eat with other people, and mess about with their food instead of eating it
- leave the table before meals are ended (often to spit the food out somewhere or make themselves sick in the toilet)
- spend all their time weighing themselves and recording all the details
- do very devious things and behave very secretively
- tell everybody that they don't have any problems, especially with their weight
- take huge amounts of exercise, often overdoing things
- wear clothes which conceal that they are in fact very thin.

IS THERE ANY TREATMENT?

At the moment we can't stop people from getting anorexia and there is a lot of argument over the best ways of treating it. However, most anorexics do get better, with only about one in three going back to having a problem.

First though, someone has to recognize that there *is* a problem, and this is usually not the person who has got it. Secondly, the person who has got it, has to be persuaded that he or she does need help. It doesn't really matter who gives the help to begin with—parent, teacher, friend. After that, the family doctor is the best person to go to, who may then ask a specialist at the hospital for more help. Usually this can be given by regular visits to hospital, but if the anorexic is very, very thin, he or she might have to stay in hospital for several weeks. This is because anorexia can be VERY dangerous. Some people die from the effects of starvation.

Mum says she read somewhere that if you put food on a very big plate it makes the anorexic think that they are eating a smaller portion than they actually are. Myself, I can't understand how people can starve themselves like that.

Ate three jam tarts with cream and a whole Yorkie after reading all this.

5th July

At last Pete seems to have found a proper girl-friend. It's Sandy (who used to go out with Randy Jo and is in the lower sixth). Kate says that her mum says that Sandy's dad is in hospital. I'm really pleased for Pete that he's found someone who likes him at last!

⑩ Whose Job is it Anyway?

6th July

It's strange not having to revise every day. Don't know what to do with myself. Dad says that Pete and I should now be doing ALL the washing-up and housework. Mum let us off during the exams. Parents shouldn't have children in the first place if they can't cope with it all.

I'm a bit scared of work experience next week. Sam's got a job with Pete unloading lorries at M & S. Wish I could work with him. That was *my* first choice. Second choice was trailing round with a barrister. Would have really liked to do this too—fancied the murder, sex and violence. John got it instead. Maybe he'll tell me all the juicy details. Actually I'm pretty angry about it. What have I ended up doing? Working as an assistant in a primary school, where nearly all the teachers are women. It's blatant sexism, though Mr Rogers said it was nothing to do with sex but just happened to work out that way. Laughable hypocrisy again.

7th July

Raining, nothing to do, fed up, miserable, hopeless. Reminds me of what I went through when I was 13. At that age I used to think I was the only one with the miseries, but then I found out that a lot of others had them too. Sometimes I would come home from school, go up to my room, and cry. I thought everyone and everything was against me, and I would have no social life or friends ever. I thought my parents didn't care, that no one cared. I would talk to my teddy or Bov, as they couldn't answer back like Pete always does. I remember Mum saying, 'It's just your age.' If only I had known how right she was. I thought I was the only person in the universe who felt like that. Everybody else was blissfully happy, could do their schoolwork, and had friends they could talk to. At school we joke about it now and compare what we all went through—but I don't feel much like laughing and joking today.

8th July

Awful day. Mum said I couldn't go out unless I cleared up my room. I'm 16 and she treats me like a child.

9th July

Better—first day at work experience. The children are really sweet but a bit much. Me and Emma couldn't step out into the playground for fear of being mobbed on all sides by a thousand 5-year-olds. One little girl jumped on me from behind. She landed flat on her face on a step and cut her lip. I didn't know what to do. There was blood everywhere. Then the lady on duty turned up and took her off to the secretary's office.

It's a real ego-booster to have thirty children looking up to you.

Also, it makes me feel good knowing I can teach them something. (So different from the constant put-down from my friends.)

10th July

Problems with the teacher I'm working for today. She started off giving me one specific thing to do. Then when she saw how much I was enjoying piddling around helping in the drawing corner, she lumbered me with a great box of pencils to sharpen. Emma's having the same problem. We both had blisters to compare at the end of the day. Also, the teacher gets angry if I get too friendly with the kids. Mind you, from the way some of them look I'm not sure I wouldn't catch something from them. Classrooms are a prime breeding spot for nits, with the children working head to head and walking around with their hair touching. You can almost see the lice crawling across. Being infested once this year is enough for me, thanks.

11th July

Sent off by Mrs Joels to buy some labels for a project. The way some shopkeepers look at people my age is insulting. This one's eyes followed me everywhere. They think we're all shoplifting vandals. Wrinklies nick things too. Since when has being young meant you're a thief, a vandal or generally something less intelligent than a piece of pasta? They're also always on about how we use bad language and are damn cheeky.

Mum's getting on my nerves more and more too. I'll ask her a simple question needing a simple answer and she'll give me a long talking to, which really gets me.

13th July

Glad to be out of the clutches of those pestering hands. Yesterday I just sat thinking 'don't touch me', but today I had to smile pleasantly while all my class kissed me goodbye and gave me cards. I enjoyed the variety of the work but think next time I'll make it clear from the start that no children will be allowed to hold on to me. At first I was so keen to fit in I didn't realize the consequences of letting one of them sit on my knee. Now I'm just relieved to be rid of the demanding little voices and the stupid teacher, who didn't even say goodbye.

Pete's in a real peck. Doesn't want me to go to parties which he's going to, even if I'm invited. Think Mum must have said something about Brenda. I told Pete it was paranoia on his part. He hates it when I use long words. He bet me I didn't know what it meant, but I told him, 'It's thinking people are getting at you when they're not.' I am a Health Freak too! He thinks he's the only know all around, but girls have brains too.

Lots of people are leaving school—for jobs, training and unemployment. I'm furious because Sheila's dad won't let her stay on to do her 'A's. He said that girls don't need to get an education as they are just going to raise a family. Neo-Victorian Fascist.

16th July

Lovely letter from Charlotte who's still having a good time in Birmingham. I miss her a lot.

Dearest Honeybunch

Hope this gets to you before you go away. If it doesn't—bloody postman's on strike. Well, how did it go? What? Ha ha your intellectual ha ha work experience ha ha again. God, I am in a mature mood tonight. It's because it's the eve of my birthday, I guess—did you? I can see you shaking your head. I am not usually like this, am I??? Well, school has finished which is a relief. Then again, I've so much work to do—two art projects and a couple of lovely essays. But I wanted to get a job. (Have you seen that advert—GET A JOB? It's pretty funky I reckon.) A job at the local pub (yes—even though I am under age)—not the one down the road, but a bike ride away. I have seen some gorgeous blokes serving behind the bar there—know what I mean?

It was great talking to you on the phone the other day. I could hardly understand what you were saying though. So if I said the wrong reply to anything it was because I couldn't hear properly and was just saying 'yes', 'no', 'it's all right for some', which I usually say to my mum and dad when I'm not listening. Hope you have a groovy time on holiday. I'm going away in a couple of weeks which should be fun.

How is your non-eating sweets, cakes and crisps going? Given up have you? I can't get through a day without at least one piece of chocolate. I'm sure it's addictive. I'm going swimming every morning to get me and my body fit. Yes—even on the morning of my birthday. Wow Char, you're fab—how doja do it?

My brother's become a real pain—constantly being silly, saying wonderful things like, 'Char you've got hairs growing out of your chin, just like mummy.' Charming boy—I hate six-year-olds. (So do I after last week's work experience.)

Well honey, I had better send this off—your bestest mate ever

Charlotte xxx

19th July

Brenda's passed her driving test. Pete thinks it's her breasts that got her through. He's a real male chauvinist pig.

Had jab at school today against tetanus. Don't need another for ten years, and no lock jaw if I cut myself. Should have had it last year, but forgot to give Mum the form to sign (scared of the needle). Had to line up with all the giggling fourth-years. 'Bet it hurts', 'Suppose I faint?', 'I feel funny already', 'Please miss can I have it another time?', 'Cor look at the size of the needle'. Don't know what the fuss was about. It only hurt if you knocked it a bit afterwards. Had a drop of polio stuff at the same time.

We've got to make our 'A' level choices tomorrow, when our sixth-form induction course ends. I haven't the faintest idea. Can't really decide before I know my exam results, can I? Pete suggested knitting, PE and French—I hope he's failed all his. Mum suggested biology, history and English and Dad suggested maths, physics and biology. My physics teacher, Miss Boil, was helpful. She asked me what I thought I wanted to do as a job in the future. I haven't really thought. I used to want to be a vet during my 'furry animal' stage. During the last ten years I've wanted to be a racing-car driver, lawyer, woman priest, accountant, computer engineer, business woman, balloonist, explorer, jet pilot, actress, poet, novelist. Now I actually have to make some kind of decision, I can't.

I put myself down for physics, maths and English, but can change it later if I want to.

20th July

School ends today. Pete and Sam and their friends are driving up to Scotland in Sam's dad's second car. Some of us hardly even have a first one—Dad's has been on its last legs for five years. I'm desperate to go—would even put up with Pete. But no no no—no from Pete, no from Sam, no from Mum and Dad. Hate Mum and Dad. I'm 16 now, and anyhow what do they think I'd get up to? Why don't they trust me? I would just have a great time—that's all. And it would be better than going to Wales with Mum, Dad and Gran.

Anyway, I couldn't really go as Marie is going to arrive from France next week. Hope we have more to say to each other than we did when I was there.

29th July

Marie's arrived, and it's not going to be easy. Pete's gone off to Scotland—sharing the driving with Sam, as he's just got his test. They set off down the road at 50 miles an hour, and screamed round the corner. Dad wondered whether he should have taken out a life insurance on Pete. Mum called him 'heartless' and burst into tears.

11 Summer Love?

1st August

Great summer holiday this:
Scribbling in the back of the car crammed between Gran and Marie
    and on the way to God knows where.
Gran's spare teeth in a plastic box nipping my neck.
Car's broken down twice already.
It's pouring with rain.
NOW stuck in a five-mile traffic jam on the motorway.
Bovril's been sick and stinks.
Marie's sulking because Pete's not coming.
I'm sulking because Marie's coming and Sam's gone with Pete.
Dad's sulking because Gran's coming.
Mum's sulking because Dad's sulking.
Gran never stops talking.

And all this for what?—two weeks in a caravan in wet and windy Wales.

Five hours later—and still not there. In fact we're not anywhere as we're lost. Mum insisted on a bit of 'culture'—a visit to Iron-bridge, full of things that happened in the Industrial Revolution. Luckily I'd done a bit about it at school. Marie was bored stiff and spent her time in the coffee bar with 'a headache'. Found her chatting up some French-speaking hunk. First words she'd said since we set out.

Dad's in a bate. Usual complaint about women lacking the 'map-reading gene'. Sexist. I'm much better than Pete at finding my way around.

2nd August

Woke snuggled cosily against the ceiling. Bright sun beaming through a chink. Bov sitting on my head by my left ear. Pee and flush of Dad in the bog. Lovely smell of Gran making tea—a steaming cup appeared at the edge of my bunk. Groan from Mum for us all to shut up please. Marie like a collapsed jelly fish in the bunk opposite.

Just one small problem—I'm on again. Wonder whether Mum and Marie (Gran must be past it?) will get it too—all of us living so close together. It's our pheromones again. They cause it—so I read—all of us starting our periods together.

Am lying in my bunk writing this and reading *Enter Tom*. Yet ANOTHER boy falling in love with his teacher. Can't see what they see in them—why can't they fall in love with me? Great not having to get up. Not so great not even being able to fart without the world knowing about it in this small space. Doesn't stop Gran though. Suppose she's got not to mind seeing that she can't control it. Privilege of the old. I couldn't get away with it. Wish I had a gas mask at this very moment—if anyone lights a match the whole caravan will explode. Will be driven to get up to get away from the smell.

Last time I farted pompous Pete *had* to notice. 'I do detect you're expelling flatus at the distal end of your digestive tract. Couldn't you have eructated instead?' As usual, he had to go on about how my fart was partly all the air I swallowed because I talked so much and partly made up of methane and hydrogen sulphide gas from the bugs in my gut working on the food I ate. All in front of Sam too. 'You're just one large walking fart, being a vegetarian and insisting on eating so many beans.' He's a real fart-arse himself—knowing all the answers to everything—but I miss him on this holiday.

3rd August

Sun, sun, sun. Marie's got all the gear—sun glasses, before-tanning creams, tanning creams of every number, after-tanning creams, beach towel—the lot. Her bikini is about as big as four mouse droppings. Mum's horrified. Keeps saying how it's cold and shouldn't Marie put a jumper on. My bikini looks like an overcoat compared with hers, and I've only got Mum's smelly old hand towel and a bottle of last year's suntan lotion.

Spent morning lying on the beach. We started with just us, and gradually became surrounded by white spotty male bodies, all eyeing Marie, making remarks, and laughing like nurds. Then Gran arrived with a deckchair, looking like a Giles granny—vast knickers and hair bulging out of a bathing cap. She plonked down next to Marie and spoilt her sexy image. Old people are really embarrassing sometimes. Not that Gran notices. She completed the picture by starting her knitting. She keeps nodding off—fell asleep in her soup last night. Gran says she can't help it—the doc says it's called narcolepsy. I say it's old age and so does Dad. Mum and Dad spent the morning in the caravan. Wonder what *they're* up to?

Marie seems different from in France. Her mum is like a real madame and is really strict with Marie. Now Marie's here she wants a mass rave up and the cinema or a disco every night. Hope I'm not going to have to put up with her wingeing and pitying herself all the time.

By evening I was knackered by the sun but still dead white. I'd borrowed Marie's number 15 sun cream. I'm scared of getting skin cancer—like on Reagan's nose. Still—this white is ridiculous. Number 10 tomorrow. Then I looked at my back in the mirror! Great red streak where I hadn't reached properly with the stuff—could even see my finger marks! Just when I wanted to start having a beautiful bronze body.

It's hard work having someone you don't know very well and don't particularly like crammed into this space. Marie said she was off for a walk before supper. Some 'walk'! When I went to get milk from the camp shop, there she was being chatted up by the greasos who were camping on the beach. Not that I'm jealous, or even fancy them, but I *would* like some kind of 'holiday romance'. Something I can tell Kate and the others about when I get back. After all, a bit of excitement is what holidays are all about. Kate always gets off with some incredibly handsome 20-year-old Porsche driver—or so she says. She lies about her age and thinks you can break all the rules on holiday.

4th August

Sun. Juggling act with Marie's sun screens today. Number 12 on most of me and number 15 on the parts which the other screens hadn't reached. Asked Marie to rub it on my back, but one of her poncy admirers flounced over, took the bottle from her and started rubbing it in. I could've sunk into the sand and disappeared with embarrassment, but it was nice at the same time. His name's Lee. He thinks it's great I'm a vegetarian, as he's a Green. He works as a lab technician in some place near New-castle. We chatted in the café while Marie disappeared in the direction of the greasos' tents.

5th August

Sun. Met Lee on the beach again. He made a rude remark as I

was spraying on some deodorant after a swim. His work's to do with a project measuring the radiation reaching earth from the sun. He's into how the chlorine from chlorofluorocarbons (the stuff that makes the spray cans spray) is damaging the layer of stuff around the earth in the upper atmosphere called 'the ozone layer'. Just one chlorine atom mucks up 10,000 ozone molecules. He seems to know everything about it, and says the ozone layer is important because it mops up ultraviolet light before it reaches the earth's surface. This ultraviolet-B light is what causes skin cancer and the more that gets through, the more skin cancer people who are out in the sun will get. Lee said the other problem is that people are sunbathing more nowadays. Luckily all the new high factor sun screens (12 to 15) help cut out the ultraviolet-B light. Most people in hot countries have always known to avoid being out in the summer sun between 11 and 3 o'clock. This is when the sun is at its strongest and can do the most harm. I was getting dead worried till Lee said skin cancer doesn't really happen until we're older. He said I should think about it now though, because if I got a bad sunburn or had too much sun it would damage my skin and increase my chances of getting skin cancer when I'm older.

Mum is going spare about Marie. She's off all the time with the boys from the tents and Mum doesn't know what to do. Must be worse when you're having to look after someone else's child. Dad was called in to be heavy. Mum took Gran and me off to the café. I swear I could hear Dad shouting even from there. Marie is red-eyed. All her beautiful make-up was smudged when we got back. Dad said there was no need for me to be smug and I'd better behave or I'd get the same treatment. Total gloom and doom in the caravan. So much for holidays. What am I going to do about seeing Lee?

6th August

Rain. Has Marie got problems. The latest is spiders. I don't like them, but Marie goes bananas. Mum says it's a 'phobia' and wishes it was a 'boy phobia'. A caravan is certainly not the place for a holiday if you don't like spiders.

We all sat round telling one another about things people hate. Dad had read that Queen Elizabeth I hated roses. Freud, the headshrink, hated travelling, and King Edward VII wouldn't let anyone mention the number '13'. Hans Christian Andersen was afraid of everything. He was so scared of fire that when he stayed in a hotel he used to sleep with a rope around him so that he could escape. He was terrified of dirt too and washed his hands 100 times a day.

Dad thinks it's all a bit silly. In his job he's always meeting people with phobias about mice, rats, wasps, fleas, lice, spiders, beetles—in fact all creepy crawlies. He's also seen people cured. What they do is first get them to look at photographs of what they hate—say, spiders. Once they can manage that, they get them to pick up a photo. Then they get them to look at the real thing, stroke it with a pencil, and then actually touch it. I wouldn't fancy going to bed with a tarantula! Gran had a friend who she called 'agoraphobic' because she couldn't go out of her house. She got treated in the same way. They took her to the door and just showed her the outside first, then took her a short distance, and then a little bit more each time she went out.

For Marie, it's not just spiders; she also has a thing about flying. Can't even bear going to the airport, let alone getting on a plane. 'Ze only time I flewed—my 'art it went boom, boom, boom, I breezed very fast, my fingers zey teeengled, my knees zey went to ze jelly, my skeen it was like a pooooool of water.'

Dad's got a phobia because there's 'a great pooooool of water' on his bed where the roof is leaking.

7th August

Rain, rain, rain. Marie and I wanted to spend the day in the café (I haven't seen Lee for two days). But we were dragged off by Mum and Dad for some 'fresh air'. Marie thinks that the 'maladie Anglais' is having picnics on the beach in freezing cold rain. We spent the rest of the day playing cards.

Another Leeless day, but it might have been him whistling at 11.30. I'm trying not to worry about my exam results.

10th August

Sun—and I've managed to see Lee at last. I'd gone with Marie to buy some insect repellant (the roll-on kind—not the aerosol) and he was in the shop. Marie had already disappeared in the direction of the tents. Lee asked if I'd come for a walk on the beach. I thought—why not? might never get the chance again. You only live once. At least here on holiday I can turn up the sexiness a bit. At home I'd just be called fresh. He may not be the most handsome guy in the world, but he's here, and he seems to like me.

We sat (well, a bit more horizontal than sitting) in a hole in the dunes, out of the wind, and told each other about our lives, though I lied about my age and tried to sound experienced. I began to wish I hadn't when things began to get a bit heavy. I wasn't sure just how far to go. I certainly didn't want to go too far. After a while, I began to feel as if it was getting out of control, and I wanted to stay in control, thank you very much. Suddenly, I noticed a distant figure. It was Dad, which brought things to a very sudden halt. Necking hasn't spoilt my feelings for Lee—though I'm not sure what he thinks of me now.

Got back to find Gran on the steps of the caravan, shaking out sand from her bri-nylon knickers covered with skidmarks.

If the article I read in *Mizz* is right—that every kiss takes three minutes off your life—I reckon I must be nearly dead by now. Feel exhausted and can't write any more tonight.

Hope Mum and Dad don't notice Marie's love bites. She was desperately trying to cover them up with make-up.

11th August

Sun, but it might as well be raining because Lee's going today. I saw him in the café. He hadn't told me he was off. He still seems to like me, took my address and promised to write.

Boring day. Don't know what to do now Lee's gone. Sunbathing's really pointless. All you do is get brown and then cover it all up because it's too cold. Anyway, people who live in hot countries have really wrinkled skin. I don't want mine to look like Gran's when I'm Mum's age. Mum asked what the matter was. Why does she want me to be happy all the time? I can't be. She isn't.

14th August

Going home tomorrow. And Marie's going back to France. The last few days have really dragged.

⑫ Romance and Results

15th August

Home to Pete. So pleased to see him, gave him a hug. He pushed me off and told me to stop being emotional, though he was obviously pleased to see me. Why do boys find it so difficult to show emotion? Hope he's more affectionate with Sandy when he sees her again. Bov's OK on emotion. She showed she was pleased to be home—slept on my bed last night. At last, no Marie, though in some ways I miss her. Especially the card games, and she was part of the 'boys' scene too.

No letter from Lee—surprise, surprise—but maybe I'm expecting too much. Even if I never see him again, he's turned me on to the idea of being a lab technician and doing something useful in life.

Sal's just back from a cheap package holiday to Spain with her girl-friend. Sal's boy-friend couldn't go because he had to work. They won't tell me the details of what they got up to. Said I was too young to know about that sort of thing yet. Must've been good though—they seem hyped up about it. I told them about my

HOLIDAY ROMANCE SURVIVAL KIT

1   Never give away something you might want back, whether it's a gold charm left to you by your grandmother, or your virginity.

2   Beware of moonlight, soft guitar music, sweet words, and cheap red wine.

3   Don't take anything back with you that you don't want. Unwanted pregnancies, VD or AIDS are not easy to get rid of.

4   If you might need them, and if you don't know the Italian, Greek, Spanish, Turkish, French or Swedish word for condoms, take them with you. If your memory is bad, you're careless, or just not good at languages—remember the 'morning after' pill. This can be used up to seventy-two hours after making love, but doesn't protect you against diseases. And you do need to get it from a doctor!

5   Never go back to the same place and expect your hulk to fall into your arms—he's probably in somebody else's.

6   Don't expect your feelings, or his, to be the same when you get back home. Holiday romances are holiday romances. One of the definitions of romance is that it's a wild and wanton exaggeration, very remote from the experiences of everyday life.

'romance' so they showed me their 'Holiday Romance Survival Kit' which they'd got from one of the newspapers. Sal said that although the books were right in saying one had to be responsible and considerate, sometimes she just wanted to have a good time. In some ways she felt that was OK, as long as she was careful. I revealed to Sal that I was the author of the 'Be Prepared' article in the school newspaper. Think she approved.

16th August

Pete got his exam results today, and managed to live up to his reputation. Two 'A's and a 'C'. He said what really gave him the piss was the 'C', as he had worked his bollocks off in chemistry but blew the practical. (He actually set his experiment on fire!) He was especially annoyed because Randy Jo got the same, and appeared to have done no work. Randy thought 'looking as if you worked' had no street cred.

Radically cool Sam sent me a postcard! which arrived today too. Goodbye Lee, welcome back Sam.

20th August

Sandy's back from her hols now. Never see Pete. Even Mum's noticed it.

22nd August

My exam results tomorrow. Mum said she'd drive me down to the school as I'd 'forgotten' to send a stamped and addressed envelope.

1 a.m.—can't sleep. Rotten having 'brainy' Pete as a brother. At least Sal understands. Sure everyone's done better than me. Anyhow, I don't really care how I've done. It's not as if me failing my exams is the end of the world. There's a lot else in life. Mum and Dad have been good about not applying pressure, but I still feel they'd like me to do well.

23rd August

Well, this is it. Crunch time in ten minutes—must get up.

Yippee! It was OK—very OK, for me anyhow. All the way there I insisted to Mum that I'd failed everything as a way of protecting myself. Couldn't face going in myself, so sent Mum instead. She came out looking furious, and I thought, 'Oh no—that's it.' Then Mum burst out laughing—3 'A's (for biology, maths and history), 2 'B's, 1 'C', and 1 'U' (for French). At least that wasn't a surprise, though Mum wanted to go for a re-mark. No way.

Kate rang and asked about my holiday. Neither of us could quite bring ourself to ask about the other's results, though I was desperate to know hers. Pete, of course, said that it was just freaky marking. Don't think he likes competition from his little sister.

Dad's really pleased. At least he doesn't think that 'good looks' is all that matters in girls, though boys seem to think different. He'd seen a survey showing that what boys most admired in girls were: (1) good looks (2) understanding (3) warmth (4) honesty (5) loyalty (6) tenderness and only (7) intelligence. Independence, forcefulness and ambition all came last. When it came to what girls admired in boys, it was still good looks at number 1. Then: (2) understanding (3) honesty (4) loyalty (5) warmth (6) intelligence. Ambition, forcefulness and independence again came low. What was really weird was that the same survey showed that what teenagers really cared about most was: (1) cruelty to animals (that would be me two years ago, but now I worry more about pollution—thanks to Lee—who still hasn't written) (2) education (3) famine (4) racial discrimination (5) unemployment and (6) nuclear war.

28th August

A lot of my friends are still away and it's starting to get boring, though I don't want the holidays to end. Everyone is surprised that I did as well as I have. Even Mary rang up to congratulate me. Generous of her as she failed three of hers. It's horrible of me, but I feel glad she did badly—she deserved to. She spends all her time out with boys. I know it's awful of me, and I know I'll probably regret it, but it's just the way I feel right now.

31st August

Looking forward to seeing all my friends and having a good gossip. Pete's worried because Sandy's dad is back in hospital with some kind of heart problem. He didn't know the right words to say to comfort Sandy.

13 Falling to Bits

1st September

Still haven't fixed my 'A' level options. Totally confusing. Why now? I hate making decisions. Seems as if the whole of the rest of my life depends on them. Back to school in three days. Can't face it. When I get fed up like this it's usually because I'm tired or bored. I looked in the mirror this morning and thought, 'God, aren't you ugly.' Then I thought how pretty everybody else is. When I'm in this mood I usually bite somebody's head off—Mum's—she makes me the maddest. She treats me as if I was a child, and makes comments and jokes that I'd make to a 3-year-old. In her eyes I'm still a little girl, but in mine I'm an adult. I feel like an adult, and I want to make my own decisions without consulting her first. Trouble is that in her day you were the age you were and that's how you felt, but nowadays you have the mind of a 20-year-old in the body of a 16-year-old. Mum thinks she's preparing me for a big bad world, but I know as much as she does about life.

2nd September

Just can't write. Totally hopeless.

4th September

Back to school today. Great to see my friends again.

5th September

Can't stand it—the house is hopping with fleas. *Pulex irritans*, Dad calls them. Twenty species attack man, and it takes one to three weeks for the eggs to hatch after being laid. At least in this country they don't carry plague, or any other nasties. I hate Bov. If only she wasn't so promiscuous. I think fleas should be counted as a sexually transmitted disease. It certainly is with her. I'm bitten all the way from my ankles to my knees, and look a real sight. Mum, Dad and Pete are all scratching. It's always worst when we get back from the summer holidays. Dad says it's because the eggs hatch out in the warm wet weather. Of course, the family with a pest control father is the last to get treated. He keeps promising to bring his spray stuff home, but it's always 'tomorrow, tomorrow'. Like my flute practice (which is why I decided to give it up).

If I could have one wish at the moment, I'd wish they'd improve the food at school. It doesn't matter how many times us vegetarians complain, nothing is ever done. I've got the girls on the school council to organize a questionnaire on what everyone eats and what they would like to eat. I think now we're in the sixth, we should have more responsibility.

6th September

Pete's still working at M & S and is loaded with dosh. He's beginning to worry about going to Nottingham. He's not so sure now he really wants to do medicine. He wishes he'd taken a year off.

I'm still faking it—trying to smile when I'm actually in a pit. Can't put the bad things out of my mind. Anyway, I've at last decided on my 'A' levels. I'm going to do sciences—maths, biology and physics. I got a 'B' for physics (so much for what Miss Boil said on my report!). And I still quite like the idea of being a lab technician, in spite of Lee not writing.

7th September

Can't face another two years of school, with the same people and the same teachers. Why doesn't anything exciting ever happen in my life?

8th September

Went round to Emma's. Not there. Her mum says Emma, Kate, Sheila and Mary—MY mates (I thought) have gone off to town. Never thought to ask me, did they? Ganging up against me. Pete says I'm being paranoic. Spent afternoon crying and talking to Bov. Got to talk to SOMEONE.

9th September

My mates came round! Turned out they were buying me a
Jimi Hendrix record yesterday because they thought it would
make me feel better. They knew I was in a pit.

We're all going through it. Kate says she's fed up with her

body. It's not that she thinks life would be any better if she was
slim, but her head would be less screwed up. If she diets, she
just puts it back on again when she stops. She can cope with not
eating till she gets her period, but after that she gets mad
cravings. She can be very strict about her eating for a day or so
and then something snaps and she stuffs her face with
chocolate, chips, sweets, anything fattening. This has emotional
effects because she feels guilty and worthless, and physical
effects like spots and headaches. She wishes she could develop
anorexia nervosa, even though she knows it is a deadly disease.
What a stupid thing to wish for.

Thank goodness I'm happy with myself today and I'm not
obese. If others aren't happy, that's their loss. Funny how moods

come and go. When Emma felt she couldn't do the work they set her at school last term, she wanted to pack the whole lot in, and leave without taking the exams. Sheila's had it crucially bad. She will have to resit some of her GCSEs at evening class, and now she's worried she won't be able to get a job. She nearly got raped and didn't get much support from her parents, and now she feels she can't talk to them about anything. During the summer, when she'd had a few drinks, she nearly decided to kill herself, like Roger Simpson at St. Joseph's School last year. Nobody realized he was depressed. He seemed to have everything going for him. He sat in his dad's car in the garage with the engine on. Really sad. Everybody felt guilty because they could've done something if they'd known. Depression can be treated, just like any other illness.

Sheila rang the Samaritans. She got their number from the local phone book. She gave it to us—said, 'You never know.' They'd helped her a lot. They'd listened to all her troubles which made her feel better. They said they got 50,000 calls a year from teenagers, so she certainly wasn't alone. They'd suggested that if she couldn't talk to her parents, she should come and see them. They're open from 8 in the morning till 10 at night, and someone is around all night to take calls. Or she could go and see her family doctor. They said they wouldn't say anything to her parents unless she wanted them to. Must be a really depressing job working at the Samaritans.

Sal came in to see me in the evening. She's very changeable. When she's got nothing better to do, she comes into my room and expects me to amuse her. She'll be nice to me and I'll tell her some of my problems, or talk to her about some boy or other that I fancy. But when she and her boy-friend come round, and I come down and watch telly or something, she tells me to go away. I've got just as much right to be there as her. More, as I live here. If I say that she starts getting nasty—telling her boy-friend everything I've told her confidentially. Then suddenly, like this evening, she expects me to be nice to her again.

Sal's boy-friend's mum works for the Samaritans. It could even have been her on the phone to Sheila. I told Sal about us all being down—Sal's been the same in her time. She'd got some gruesome facts from her boy-friend's mum.

- suicidal thoughts are much more common than threats or actual attempts, and about 1 in 20 boys and about 1 in 10 girls have suicidal thoughts at one time or another.
- actual suicide is rare before the age of 14. About 5,000 teenagers per year attempt suicide, but most of them don't actually want to kill themselves. There are about 120 suicide deaths a year in England and Wales in this age group, and many of these teenagers don't mean to kill themselves either.
- among all the attempted and actual suicides, there is a definite reason in 2 out of 3 cases, and no clear reason for the others.
- the main reasons for suicidal thoughts and attempts are: trouble with parents, broken homes, school work, worries about exam failure, fear of unemployment, and relationship problems with a boy or girl-friend. In some cases it is a way of getting away from intolerable stress, and letting other people know how unhappy they are.
- main feelings that occur before some of the attempts are: anger, feeling lonely or unwanted, worries about the future, and—if depressed as well—feelings of hopelessness.

Sal said that when her friend was very depressed a few years ago, she became stroppy, bad-tempered, quiet and withdrawn; she was always tired, kept bursting into tears, and didn't want to be with anyone. She saw her family doctor and used up all his supply of Kleenex. He didn't seem to mind—he had boxes of them everywhere. He arranged for her to see a sympathetic person called a counsellor, and said that if that didn't work she might need some tablets.

None of this sounded like me. When I get depressed I listen to Jimi Hendrix records—which Pete says drives HIM to murderous rather than suicidal thoughts. I also cope by ringing up a friend and having a long natter—that usually cheers me up, by going out with my mates, or reading a book. If I can't do any of those, I sulk till someone notices. Then I have a good moan and that makes me feel better too.

I suppose feelings of sadness are just part of growing up. It's only if they go on for a long time—or get very bad—that one should worry. If mine got very bad, I'd realize I was ill and would go and get some help.

12th September

We're all into words. Why are words so important I wonder? Why do they change, like fashions?

Sixties
Groovy, fab, ciao, happening, pad, boutiques, far OUT, gear, too good, way out, weird.

Seventies
Hassle, no problem, take care, situation, laid back, zoned, smashed, over the top (OTT), male chauvinist pig (MCP), scene, relate, being INTO something, not my bag, check it out, guy, heavy, trendy, great.

Smart cockney
Know what I mean, bleedin', bloke, dosh, OK mate, right, triffic, down the boozer, ta, dodgy, a right Brian.

Drug street slang, old and new
Crack, grass, high, trip, billy whizz, speed, blow, ganja, uppers, amphet, snow, coke, smack, henry, skag, gear, score, buzz, ecstasy.

For those into sex
Copulation, intercourse, fucking, shafting, shagging, bonking, making love, having it off, screwing, making it, doing it, squelching.

Yuppy talk
Designer, divine, bliss, anything in French, frock, darling, filofax, fab, too too, totally, the market, upmarket, downmarket.

Street cred
It sucks, dude, bad, wicked, yo, sweet, Babylon, def, casual, crucial, dick, ruination, mellow.

Media, media
Cool, classic, style, hip, key, modern, directional, holistic.

God, what do I need to be depressed about—it's ridiculous:

* I have lots of really nice friends
* I do look somewhat better than a dish-rag
* hardly anyone is REALLY happy at the moment—they just kind of make out they are
* Bov loves me
* my exam results weren't half bad
* my parents really do care about me, even if we do quarrel quite a bit
* I've got an ace brother
* I'm better shaped than a balloon
* Sam speaks to me occasionally
* what more could I want?

Even if I don't feel totally part of the 'in' crowd and absolutely 'with it'—it doesn't matter. Sal says nobody feels like this anyhow. I bet that the future is going to be absolutely wicked.

14 Getting it Together

16th September

Our first day at the Keep Fit club at the local pool. The Samaritans put Sheila on to it. Never dared go on my own but now we're all going. We did a fitness test before starting and had to answer some questions:

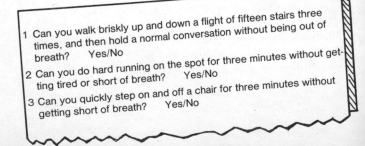

1 Can you walk briskly up and down a flight of fifteen stairs three times, and then hold a normal conversation without being out of breath? Yes/No

2 Can you do hard running on the spot for three minutes without getting tired or short of breath? Yes/No

3 Can you quickly step on and off a chair for three minutes without getting short of breath? Yes/No

4 Can you put your hands flat on the ground with your knees straight?   Yes/No

5 How many 'press-ups' can you do?
   0–5   5–10   10–15   15–20

Then they tested us. They told me I was good on stamina and suppleness but awful on strength. I only managed three press-ups. Bit embarrassing as I had said on the questionnaire I could do 10–15. We were lectured by a Russian athlete-type woman who must have been taking male hormones on her cornflakes for the last ten years—she was all hairy and muscle-bound—on the golden rules of exercise:

1 Get moving—find more active ways of doing the things you usually do, like running upstairs instead of walking.

2 Get fit gradually—it takes time. Make yourself sweaty and out of breath but not uncomfortable.

3 Exercise regularly—get into a routine.

4 Keep it up—you can't 'store up' fitness.

5 Enjoy it—make sure the activities are ones you like and can do regularly.

We must have been a sight—sitting in the sauna after an hour on the machines. All sweat and flesh, except for Kate who still looks as if she's come from a Third World disaster area. I enjoyed it. It's very sociable and a real laugh—all of us looking so gross. Kate was there trying to do away with the two kilos of what's left of her body. Sheila was there because of the Samaritans and because she's not happy with her job. She wishes she was still at school, and we wish we had her money. She thought that she would find all the jumping around and being womanhandled by Russian athletes even more depressing—but actually she's much better. Mary was there because she wants to keep her body supple and in shape for the boys, and Emma thinks that if she looks good she's nicer to people.

Nobody there liked us because they're all fat, flabby, and forty and think we're taking the piss out of them. I don't somehow think any of us will be competing in the next Olympics!

17th September

Hardly made it out of bed this morning. Don't know how I got to school today. I ache in places I didn't know existed let alone had muscles in.

20th September

Am I perverse or perverted? I think I'm becoming a 'Fitness Freak'. I haven't really thought about sport since I twisted my ankle in the 400 metres (when I was 13). Now I'm in the lower sixth where my teachers tell me I don't *have* to do it—I *want* to. But I don't want to do weedy little girls' sports like rounders and netball—boring, tedious, and going on for only three seconds at a time because of too many rules. I want to do violent sports like rugby—rampaging round the field getting really dirty, and smashing people into the ground, and swimming around in the mud. Then going off and getting pink and clean in a shower and feeling really good afterwards. Where can girls play rugby, except at posh schools costing £10,000 a year? I wonder why blokes like team sports and seem more competitive than women? Must be something to do with their upbringing. I like competing if I win—it used to be the only thing that made me run. Otherwise I found it dead boring.

Pete's a pain at the moment, letting everyone down. He thinks he's 'in love' with Sandy. I think he's being stupid. He promised to come with me and Kate to the late night cinema yesterday. Mum said we couldn't go otherwise, in case we got attacked. I sometimes think Mum is being overprotective. Just because I'm a girl she thinks I'm going to get mugged or raped. Pete was allowed out at night at my age. Then Sandy rang and asked Pete to go to the pub, and he went. He's not going to have any friends left when it finishes between him and Sandy. He keeps letting them down. Kate and I told him girls hate boys who are doormats. Pete's acting like a member of a religious cult. I don't think it's love—I think it's worship.

23rd September

A session on the torture rack again but I'm definitely getting fitter. We were lectured again by the hairy-bottomed monster, this week on the exercise value of the different sports:

Walking—great for stamina but not so good for suppleness and strength. For all-round fitness, you need another sport as well.

Swimming—excellent for strength, suppleness and stamina, especially if you use various strokes.

Cycling—great for stamina and leg strength, but not so hot on suppleness.

Jogging and running—a fun-free and quick way to get fit. Good for stamina but not so good for suppleness.

Badminton—fun even for beginners. Good for stamina, flexibility and strength.

Tennis—fun and sociable, and good all-round exercise.

Squash—very exercising, providing good all-round activity. Warm up before you start.

Team games—great for stamina and strength, and pretty good for suppleness. You don't have to be good to play.

Weight training—helps tone up your body and keep you slim and supple.

It seems you have to do an awful lot of exercise to work off the calories you put on by just drinking one pint of pasteurized milk. To do that, I would have to:

    walk for 76 minutes
    swim for 60 minutes
    walk fast for 54 minutes
    play badminton for 48 minutes
    run slowly for 47 minutes
    cycle for 46 minutes
    play tennis or do aerobics for 42 minutes
    run fast or swim fast for 32 minutes
    play squash for 22 minutes.

Pete said that making love was the equivalent exercise of running a mile. He should know. Suppose it must depend on how you do it though.

We did weight-lifting this week. I think the weights I lifted weighed more than Kate. Kate herself looked like a bent beanpole holding up Big Ben. Sheila's flagging. She thinks horse riding is more her style. She likes the feeling of power, and being taller and looking down on people. She also loves the romantic image, but knows the real thing's different—smelly and sweaty with a lot of what she refers to as 'mucking out'.

24th September

Beginning to get upset again about Lee not writing and Sam not
taking any notice of me. Anyway, Sam's about to disappear from
my life. He's off to work his way round the world. He certainly
won't be interested in ME after adventures in hot countries filled
with glamorous, sexy women. There's too much pressure
nowadays over having a boy-friend. Everyone seems to expect
you to and when you don't, you begin to wonder what's wrong.
I'm beginning to lose my confidence. It starts with one thing,
like whether I've got any friends, and goes on to another, my
looks, my clothes. Everything begins to crumble. I'm always
comparing myself with my friends. Sometimes I want to break
out and be original but I can't. How can I explain it? There are
times when I would like to buy something that other people
would call unfashionable but that I like. It's at times like this that
I really appreciate Pete being around. He's like having an extra
friend, and it gives me a good feeling of security.

25th September

Bicycling to school's more fun now I'm fitter. I beat speedy
Winston up the hill today. The good thing about cycling is that if
you're not feeling competitive you can go at your own speed,
and see things you don't see otherwise. The bad thing is the
danger I suppose. I'd wear a crash helmet if it didn't make me
feel such a dick. I still think the only way they'll get people to
wear them is by making it compulsory.

26th September

Pete's out with Sandy again. He's meant to be getting things
ready for university but seems to have a one-track mind. A
whole gang of them are going to a pop concert. They had a long
pep talk from Sam's dad about the dangers of drugs. He said the
police and the pushers were sure to be out in force—and not to
expect him to come and bail them out if they got into trouble. As
usual—I'm not allowed to go.

27th September

I've lost the key of my cycle lock, so I left my bike at school and walked.

The pop concert trip nearly ended in disaster—with them all in jail. Turned out Sam's dad—after all his lectures, and unknown to them—had forgotten to take his medical bag, containing drugs like heroin and morphine, out of the boot of the car. The police had stopped them near the concert for a routine check. The sniffer dogs were just about to start in when a psychedelic van whizzed past and got stopped and searched instead. It wasn't till they got back, they realized what a near miss it had been! Pete said that there were dealers sidling up all the time, trying to sell crack, cheap. He wanted to smash their faces in.

28th September

Still no bike, but I have the key. Found it this evening in Bov's basket. How did it get *there*?

29th September

Bike, key and lock all together at last. Collected bike from school in spite of the fact it's Saturday. Pete tore himself away from Sandy to drive me down in Dad's car.

All my pals are coming round this evening for a 'gathering'. (No, Mum—it's *not* a party.)

30th September

Was struggling out of bed to go to Keep Fit club—aerobics this week—when sudden scream of anger from Mum. She's cracked at last. Is this the end of the 'rave up' age?

Why was the milk out of the fridge?
Why was there no bread left?
Why had all the lights been left on downstairs?
Why was the toilet blocked with paper?
Why was the kitchen floor covered with crisps?
Why had the apple pie that was for Sunday lunch been eaten?
Why did everyone use the ice-cubes and put the ice-cube tray back empty?
Why had three glasses been smashed?
Why did no one ever change the bog rolls?
Why did no one ever clean out Pinko's cage?
Why had no one fed the cat?
Why was the sink full of washing up?
Why did no one ever put their own dirty washing into the machine?
Why was the bottle of Jamieson's whisky all drunk?
Why was there a cigarette burn on the sofa?
Why was the back door left unlocked?
Why were there three strange bicycles in the hall?
Why was this house such a pigsty?

Pete didn't seem to think there was a problem—which didn't help Mum's mood. Dad stayed out of the fray and in bed most of the day.

Never made it to aerobics, unless you count clearing up at home as aerobic exercise. Mum said I'm not missing anything as long as I take *some* exercise and today she'd rather it was at home—thank you very much.

Death, Dreads and Drama

1st October

Pete's in the dumps, getting at me in particular and the world in general. He referred to the human race as 'a foul genetic mistake'. Told *me* to 'grow up'. Informed me that I seemed to think that all there was to being mature was being aged 16, being able to make love legally and get married, making decisions about 'A' level choices, being able to have a conversation of more than three sentences, and *now* being allowed to stay out till midnight by Mum and Dad. He seems to think that his extra two years' experience makes all the difference. He's so bloody patronizing. Old 'know all' doesn't even seem to know about women maturing earlier than men.

Anyhow, he and Sandy are pathetic—going around together like an old married couple. I suppose it's because he's about to go off to university.

2nd October

SANDY'S DAD HAS DIED. He had another really bad heart attack at work yesterday. He was rushed off to the hospital but was DEAD when he got there. Pete doesn't know what to do. Whether to ring up, whether to go to the hospital, whether to go and see Sandy at home, what to say to her and her mum. Mum says he must go and see her. There's nothing worse than people avoiding you when disaster happens. That's what friends are for—to be there. She said it is bound to be difficult but emotions are something you have to face up to.

Pete came back later. He said Sandy had cried a lot but had been really pleased he'd come. Him just being there had helped her, even though it was a bit awkward at first. Sandy doesn't seem to be able to believe it's happened. She still expects her dad to walk in at any moment. Pete wants to talk about it. It feels so different from when Jason's dad died last year. Pete had found Jason in the pub the same evening, as though nothing had happened. Strange, the different reactions to death.

3rd October

Hate the idea of Mum and Dad dying. It really frightens me. Don't think I slept all night, worrying.

Pete went to the funeral. He's convinced they are a good thing. Not that he'd enjoyed it, but being there was like being able to say 'goodbye'. He thought that Mum had been wrong, not letting us go to Grandad's funeral for fear of upsetting us. Even Sandy's younger brother, aged 5, had been at the cremation. I think Pete's right because I still don't quite feel Grandad's gone. His was a heart attack too. I keep seeing people who look like him, and my heart sort of sinks each time. In spite of all the sadness, Pete looked a real laugh going off in Dad's dark suit, Sam's too-big black shoes, and awful Uncle Bob's black tie. He looked like Charlie Chaplin.

Pete's got himself a donor card. He doesn't want to be

flattened by a passing car without being useful to the human race. There are hundreds of people waiting for kidney transplants, corneal transplants and heart transplants (and me for a brain transplant, he says). Once he's dead, he doesn't care what happens to his body. He gets angry with me when I say I don't want to have surgeons arranging for bits of me to be walking about inside other people when I die.

Couldn't sleep. Came down at 2 a.m. to make Ovaltine, and found a convulsed Pete listening to the phone. He couldn't sleep either (he called it 'insomnia') and was trying all these numbers he'd found in a magazine. So far he'd phoned for information on:

What is an orgasm?

Masturbation—the facts

Is it wrong for me to dream about sex?

Can love be just lust?

The numbers had all been engaged. Now I know what insomniacs do at 2 a.m. All Pete could get through to was 'Girls' Bodies'. Couldn't think why he was laughing till I rang 'Boys' Bodies' and discovered. A disembodied voice told me of all the hidden treasures I could find inside boys' boxer shorts. I'm not sure what Dad will say about the telephone bill if I do this every night!

4th October

Exhausted. Pete insists that *he's* like Napoleon, Margaret Thatcher and Churchill, and can manage on four hours' sleep a night. Hadn't noticed this myself—especially on Sunday mornings when he stays in bed till lunchtime.

Pete had another go at Dad about smoking today. It worries him that Dad might get cancer or have a heart attack. At least he's not smoking as many as he used to.

I don't think I'll have any more arguments with my parents. What if they died suddenly and I was never able to make it up to them. I would feel that it had been my fault, and that God or whoever was punishing me and teaching me a lesson. Couldn't get to sleep for hours, for the second night running.

5th October

Pete's gone. He didn't want to go, with Sandy feeling so sad, but his term starts today. Mum drove him up to Nottingham. I miss him already. Now I'm the only one left at home.

9th October

Sandy came round. I was terrified I might giggle out of nervousness so I gave her a big hug. She burst into tears and I knew I was going to sob too. She's having to be strong, and try not to cry in front of her mum. Being the eldest, she feels she has to be responsible and support her. She said she keeps wondering what she's done wrong in life to deserve this. She goes over it again and again.

10th October

Got smashed by Emma at squash today, but it was a good game. Sandy's dad's death has made us all morbid. While banging around the squash court, Kate told me that she had had a sister who died when Kate was 5. She's never talked about it before, partly because her parents had been so awful. They'd never explained to her what had happened, and now tried to pretend that her sister had never existed. She'd gone through sheer hell when it happened, and had felt totally and utterly depressed. No one could cheer her up, no one could understand what she was going through. Her parents had said, 'Time will heal'. Although that was true, it had been the last thing she had wanted to hear then. She remembered one day when one of her friends had tickled her to cheer her up. Instead of laughing, like she usually did, she had burst into tears, and everyone had felt embarrassed.

11th October

Sandy's back at school. We're trying to be really nice to her, and really considerate, but some people don't know how.

12th October

It's just like when I had my exams. I'm not sleeping a wink at night. Mum's sympathetic and says lots of things can cause it, like anxiety, stress, depression, overwork, sadness at someone dying. Dad says that most people who think they haven't slept a wink have been found in experiments to actually go to sleep twenty minutes after going to bed, and then sleep for a good six hours. Trouble is, that's not the way it feels to me. I felt as though I lay awake all last night, worrying I was not going to get to sleep.

14th October

Still not sleeping properly. Mum said she'd find me something to read about insomnia, and that sleeping tablets were certainly NOT the answer as they are all addictive.

At least I've got Bov to keep me company, though Mum doesn't like her sleeping on my bed. Bov knows it. If Mum comes in at night, she's under the bed in a flash. Bov and I really understand one another. She never answers me back, unlike some people in this house. She's been with me for four years now. I sometimes wonder whether I'd mind her dying more than a human.

15th October

Terrible noises last night. Doesn't help my sleep problem, being scared to death. I decided it was Dad snoring, till I looked in the garden this morning. Bov's killed Pinko. I'm going to kill Bov next time I see her. Why can't cats be vegetarians?

Pinko went alongside the other eight graves—two hamsters, three rabbits, a mouse, a gerbil and Gran's budgy. I'll have to give up looking after animals. Care was needed with the grave digging as I wasn't sure what else I might come across. I hope cemeteries are more organized. Personally, I don't fancy being charcoal grilled and ending up as a little pile of grey ashes like Sandy's dad. I want to go into the ground whole—like Pinko. Dad disagrees and thinks that it is ridiculous using large parts of the countryside for burying the dead. He said it's much healthier and nicer to be cremated. Still, at least we have the choice!

16th October

At last Mum's got the stuff on how to sleep. It was in the Sunday paper. (Thought for the Day: 'Does everybody tear the cardboard roll of the toilet paper and use it when the paper has run out? If the answer is 'yes', then why don't they make it softer so it doesn't hurt one's bum so much?')

TIPS FOR NON-SLEEPERS

The bit of your body which most needs sleep is your brain. Everything from your neck down can do without it, provided it gets regular rest and food.

Even your brain, on average, only needs six hours' sleep a night, but this does vary from person to person. There appear to be two main kinds of 'sleep'—'vital' or 'deep' sleep and 'optional', 'light' or 'rapid eye movement' (because your eyes move rapidly backwards and forwards behind your closed eyelids) sleep. The second kind of sleep is when you dream, the first kind is the kind that revitalizes your brain. Short sleepers are able to miss out on 'optional' sleep but not on 'vital' sleep. Feelings of 'sleepiness' are what finally tell us whether we are getting enough sleep or not.

Some things to do:

1 Accept that *whatever* sleep you can get is going to be really enjoyable.
2 Try and go to bed at a regular time, and set an alarm so that you don't get anxious about waking up on time.
3 Don't indulge in weekend sleep binges.
4 Try relaxation exercises, or a brisk walk, in the hour or so before bed.
5 Don't indulge in heavy meals, alcohol, tea or coffee (unless decaffeinated) just before going to bed.
6 It's worth trying a glass of warm milk, Ovaltine or Horlicks.
7 Make sure your mattress and pillows are comfortable and the bedroom is not too hot or cold.
8 Pee before going to sleep.
9 If you can't get to sleep—don't toss and turn—get up and go and do something in another room. You don't want to associate your bedroom with sleeplessness.
10 Try relaxation tapes that are available in some shops.

Oh, well—can but try.

🔢 Food, Glorious Food

17th October

Something had changed when I woke up this morning. I'd slept! Waking was like swimming to the surface of a deep dark pool—up and up. Maybe it's because I think I just might have a boy-friend, at least I hope I have. I'll wait before I write his name down—it's such an embarrassing name and things might go wrong.

18th October

Lost my bike lock today but I've still got the key. Mum says I've got to buy a combination lock, and it's got to come out of my pocket-money.

19th October

My wish about school food has come true, or maybe it's POWER at last. Our 'questionnaire' has worked. The school's into 'NEW-LOOK, HEALTHY EATING', with a typical, massive 'Let's all do this together' type programme. Gym, geography, social studies, sports, a healthy eating 'word search' in the school

F	W	H	O	L	E	M	E	A	L	B	B	D	P
N	V	O	T	Z	N	P	E	A	S	A	R	O	C
U	L	E	N	T	I	L	S	F	A	N	O	U	E
N	K	T	G	O	T	F	A	P	P	T	W	G	L
S	C	P	C	E	U	F	I	S	H	A	N	N	E
A	H	U	E	Q	T	L	C	B	U	A	B	B	K
T	O	L	P	A	B	A	F	S	R	N	R	O	Y
U	N	L	E	W	R	N	B	O	I	E	E	T	C
R	L	E	Q	R	K	U	E	L	C	L	A	T	R
A	A	T	O	M	A	T	O	C	E	D	D	L	I
T	F	T	D	A	P	O	T	A	T	O	P	N	S
E	T	U	H	T	P	L	U	M	S	M	I	N	K
D	E	C	A	Z	L	C	C	E	R	E	A	L	U
A	K	E	L	P	E	K	I	L	S	E	U	M	T

magazine—even the dinner ladies are involved. Anyhow, they said they're fed up with making custard and jam pudding. The boys on the school council hate us. They've been to see the head. They even arranged for the local chip van to visit at 12.30. Maybe it's because it sells fags—one at a time—as well. Seems that smoking and unhealthy diets go together.

I'm really proud of our survey. We got the whole sixth form to think out the questions, give out the questionnaire, and analyse it on the computer. Only blot on the landscape was the one we gave to the staff. They won't let us analyse that—will they?

ANALYSIS OF 'HEALTHY EATING' QUESTIONNAIRE

Question 1

(a) Do you think the food provided by the school is healthy?
Yes—40% No—60%
(b) Do you consider the food you eat at home is healthy?
Yes—80% No—20%

Question 2

What are your favourite foods?

FAVOURITE FOODS

Question 3

Are your favourite foods available at school?
Yes—20% No—80%

Question 4

How often do you eat chips?

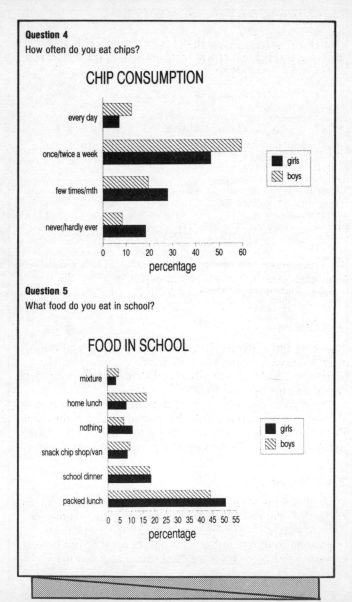

CHIP CONSUMPTION

Question 5

What food do you eat in school?

FOOD IN SCHOOL

Other Comments You Have about Health and Food in School

Don't eat the food.
They shouldn't let local shops sell fags.
What about us vegetarians? Let's have more variety—instead of just salad and a lump of cheddar cheese.
Can we have more chips please?
Raise the age you can buy fags to 18.
Why only white rolls?
More choice please—what about Indian and Chinese foods?
Why was Doreen's toe-nail in my salad?
Lots of fruit but no tarantulas please.
Why do all dinner ladies look like jam rolls?
Unbruised apples please.
Less lumps in the custard please.
Get someone to turn the water into beer.
Tidying the school up might help.
Cut out the grease!
Why can't we have more West Indian food, man?

Glad it's worked. We now have baked potatoes, wholemeal rolls, vast salads of every variety, and nice fresh fruit. Not thinner dinner ladies though! They still look like jam rolls.

21st October

OK—his name is 'Willie'. He's 1.65 metres tall, blond haired, very attractive, in the upper sixth, wears really cool shirts, smells great and apparently is a good kisser and dancer, though Sandy says he 'gets around a bit'.

Thank goodness Pete's away and doesn't know about him or the remarks would start. Willie has started coming to the Sports Centre on Sundays and we walk home together, but my friends are always with us. He says he'll help me baby-sit on Tuesday.

23rd October

'Thought for the Month'—I HATE MEN. They only think of one thing. I got Mum and Dad's permission for Willie to come and baby-sit with me at Mrs Smith's. Dad gave me a lecture on 'reputation' and stuff. Because I'm the youngest he can be very protective too. Anyway, Willie came round and after the children had gone to sleep we sat kissing for quite a long time. Then he pushed me on to the floor and asked me to have sex with him! I said 'NO'—though deep down I quite wanted to. I really fancied him, but I've only known him for two weeks. He kept on and on about it, but I still said 'NO'. He asked me, 'Why not?' I told him that it wasn't that I was scared, but that I'd never done it before, wasn't about to now, and at my age didn't relish the idea of getting pregnant. He gave me some bull about boys under the age of 18 not being able to get a girl pregnant—he must have thought I was really thick. He can't have read my ace (anonymous) article on contraception in the school newspaper. He must know the facts—he's been to the same sex education classes at school as I have. Most boys have active sperms at 13. He went on to tell me he wouldn't pack me in, and that he really loved me. Yeah, I thought, keep talking. But I wasn't going to give in, and in the end he left.

After he'd gone, I felt pretty cross. Being a virgin does mean something to me. I'm not just going to throw it away with ANYONE.

25th October

Yesterday Willie got his sister to phone and tell me that he didn't want to go out with me any more. I didn't feel upset. I kind of knew he'd do something like that. I was just really angry he hadn't had the guts to tell me to my face. At school now he's spreading rumours that I'm tight and can't kiss, and that he raped me. Personally I think he's stupid to say he raped me. He could get into a lot of trouble, and I can't imagine his friends being impressed. Boys like that just aren't worth knowing.

I told Mary a bit about it—though not the juicy details! My friends have nicknamed him 'Mini Willie'. They say he's probably got his big muscles—not because he ate the right foods and did the right exercises—but because he used anabolic steroids. Like Ben Johnson in the Olympics. Anabolic steroids give you 'deformed genitals'. Very funny thought.

26th October

No lock, no bike now—just a key. Daren't tell Mum as I never got round to buying the combination lock. Just said I felt like a walk. 'It's good exercise, Mum.'

Nurd at school, who's self-appointed leader of the 'chip and fag' gang, came up to me in the common room and said, 'I don't believe what you say about fatty foods giving you a heart attack when you're older. My grandad is 85 and has always eaten lots of greasy food, and smoked twenty fags a day.' I told him to clean out his ears. What I had said was not that fatty foods and smoking WILL give you a heart attack, but that eating fatty foods and smoking *makes you much more likely* to get a heart attack.

I thought Mum would have a heart attack when I got back and told her about the bike. But she already knew! How do they always know before you even tell them? Another thing that must come with 'maturity'.

🔟⁷ An Aid to AIDS

2nd November

Relief. Half-term this week. It's given me time to recover. What is it about me and boys?

5th November

Nobody's having fireworks this year. Too many accidents last year, and anyway Dad says fireworks cost too much. I'm disappointed. Bet we'd have them if Pete was here. His accident a few years ago hasn't put him off what he calls 'being a pyromaniac'. Sounds a bit like being a hypochondriac.

We all went to the public fireworks in the park instead. Much better fireworks, but I hate the bangs, and I had mud up to my waist when I got home. There was jazz, and hot dogs—but also crying babies and smoke.

I spotted John, with Charlie—both lit up by one of the fireworks. I hadn't set eyes on Charlie for five months! I nudged Kate—who dropped her toffee apple in the mud, and a dog ate it. I didn't think they'd seen us, then I heard John shouting my name. Charlie didn't seem to want to look at me and kept scuffing his shoes on the ground. He explained that he'd lost my phone number, and that HE was waiting for ME to phone HIM. He'd been too shy to ask John for it, in case I didn't want to see him again. I scrawled my number with Kate's eye-liner on the back of my new copy of *Just Seventeen*, and told him not to lose it this time.

6th November

The excitements of yesterday made me completely forget what was happening today. A quiffy doctor at assembly gave the whole sixth form a questionnaire. She said she wanted to know what we knew and felt about AIDS. I thought it would be all about who I was going out with. Everybody else scribbled away, so I thought they must all be doing amazing things when I wasn't even going out with anyone—(yet?)

Sita Beegam's parents wouldn't let her fill it in. She's really nice, but she's not allowed to do anything with us. She isn't allowed out in the evenings at all, and her parents won't even allow her to attend 'Personal Guidance' lessons, let alone the school Christmas party. Although Sita knows her parents do it because they were brought up that way, and they think it is best for her too—she doesn't think they understand what it is like nowadays. How is she meant to learn about relationships and sex and stuff? Her parents are even suggesting that they will arrange who she marries when she is old enough. At least they've allowed her to stay on and do her 'A' levels.

WHAT DO YOU KNOW ABOUT AIDS?

PLEASE FILL IN THIS QUESTIONNAIRE.
The answers will be given to you later

How old are you?   . . .years. . . .months
Which sex are you?   male   female

- 1   What does A. . . . . . . .I. . . . . . .D. . . . . .S. . . . . . .stand for?

- 2   What causes AIDS?

- 3   What does H. . . .I. . . .V. . . .stand for?

- 4   When was AIDS first discovered?

          1950-1960?
          1960-1970?
          1970-1980?
          After 1980?

- 5   How and where did it start?

- 6   Roughly how many people in this country have the AIDS disease?

          1000
          2000
          5000
          10,000

- 7   Roughly how many people in this country have already died from AIDS?

          50
          700
          1200
          4800
          12,500

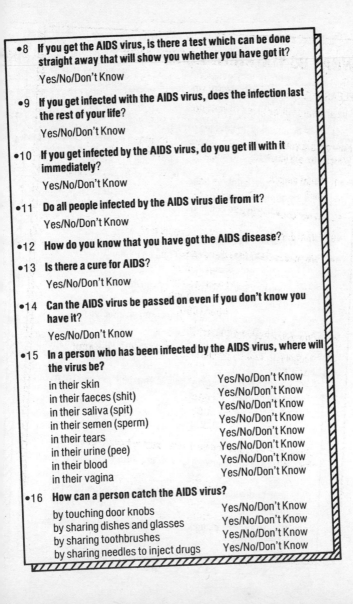

• 8 **If you get the AIDS virus, is there a test which can be done straight away that will show you whether you have got it?**

Yes/No/Don't Know

• 9 **If you get infected with the AIDS virus, does the infection last the rest of your life?**

Yes/No/Don't Know

• 10 **If you get infected by the AIDS virus, do you get ill with it immediately?**

Yes/No/Don't Know

• 11 **Do all people infected by the AIDS virus die from it?**

Yes/No/Don't Know

• 12 **How do you know that you have got the AIDS disease?**

• 13 **Is there a cure for AIDS?**

Yes/No/Don't Know

• 14 **Can the AIDS virus be passed on even if you don't know you have it?**

Yes/No/Don't Know

• 15 **In a person who has been infected by the AIDS virus, where will the virus be?**

in their skin	Yes/No/Don't Know
in their faeces (shit)	Yes/No/Don't Know
in their saliva (spit)	Yes/No/Don't Know
in their semen (sperm)	Yes/No/Don't Know
in their tears	Yes/No/Don't Know
in their urine (pee)	Yes/No/Don't Know
in their blood	Yes/No/Don't Know
in their vagina	Yes/No/Don't Know

• 16 **How can a person catch the AIDS virus?**

by touching door knobs	Yes/No/Don't Know
by sharing dishes and glasses	Yes/No/Don't Know
by sharing toothbrushes	Yes/No/Don't Know
by sharing needles to inject drugs	Yes/No/Don't Know

by using lavatory seats Yes/No/Don't Know
by giving the 'kiss of life' Yes/No/Don't Know
by wet (french) kissing Yes/No/Don't Know
by droplets of saliva Yes/No/Don't Know
by anal intercourse Yes/No/Don't Know
by holding hands Yes/No/Don't Know
by touching an infected person's
 blood Yes/No/Don't Know
by blood transfusion Yes/No/Don't Know
by head lice Yes/No/Don't Know
by mother to unborn baby Yes/No/Don't Know
by drinking breast milk Yes/No/Don't Know
by sneezing and coughing Yes/No/Don't Know
by vaginal intercourse Yes/No/Don't Know

•17 When having sex can:

a man catch the AIDS virus from an infected man?
Yes/No/Don't Know

a man catch the AIDS virus from an infected woman?
Yes/No/Don't Know

a woman catch the AIDS virus from an infected man?
Yes/No/Don't Know

a woman catch the AIDS virus from an infected woman?
Yes/No/Don't Know

•18 Give the three groups of people you think are most at risk of catching the AIDS virus:

a) . . . .
b) . . . .
c) . . . .

•19 Which of the following kills off the AIDS virus outside the body?

heat Yes/No/Don't Know
soap and water Yes/No/Don't Know
disinfectants Yes/No/Don't Know

•20 If you have sex using a condom, does it protect you against getting AIDS?

Yes/No/Don't Know

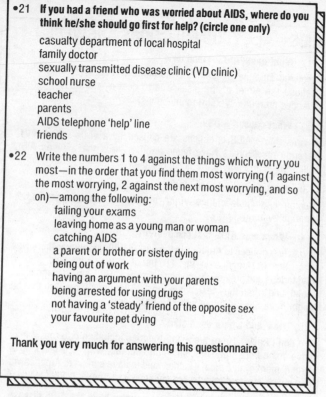

•21 **If you had a friend who was worried about AIDS, where do you think he/she should go first for help? (circle one only)**

casualty department of local hospital
family doctor
sexually transmitted disease clinic (VD clinic)
school nurse
teacher
parents
AIDS telephone 'help' line
friends

•22 Write the numbers 1 to 4 against the things which worry you most—in the order that you find them most worrying (1 against the most worrying, 2 against the next most worrying, and so on)—among the following:
failing your exams
leaving home as a young man or woman
catching AIDS
a parent or brother or sister dying
being out of work
having an argument with your parents
being arrested for using drugs
not having a 'steady' friend of the opposite sex
your favourite pet dying

Thank you very much for answering this questionnaire

What a sweat filling this in—sure I got half the answers wrong.

7th November

Think Charlie must have lost my phone number again. No way I'm going to phone him.

8th November

AIDS again at school today. The teachers gave us the answers—and there will be more answers tomorrow. They're obsessed.

AIDS—ALL YOUR QUESTIONS ANSWERED

(1) What does 'AIDS' stand for?

'Acquired Immune Deficiency Syndrome'. It was given this name because the effect of the disease is to destroy the body's normal defences (immune system) to infections.

(2) What causes AIDS?

A virus. Most AIDS infections are caused by a virus called HIV1. Recently researchers have found another virus that causes AIDS called HIV2, and others are being discovered.

(3) What does 'HIV' stand for?

'Human Immunodeficiency Virus' because it affects the body's immune system.

(4) When was AIDS first discovered?

It was first noticed in America in the early 1980s. However there was one case in America in the 1970s of a boy who died from a mysterious and previously unknown disease. They saved some of his blood, and when they tested it in the 1980s they discovered that he might have been infected with the AIDS virus.

(5) How and where did it start?

We don't know. There are many theories including one that it may have come from a person coming into contact with a certain kind of 'green' monkey in Africa. It is then said to have spread to America via one airline steward who had many sexual partners.

(6) How many new people in this country have the AIDS disease each year?

The new cases each year are:

```
1984— 77
1985—160
1986—305
1987—649
1988—539
```

(7) How many of these people had died from AIDS by the end of 1988?

Of the 77 new cases in 1984—74 are dead
Of the 160 new cases in 1985—135 are dead
Of the 305 new cases in 1986—243 are dead
Of the 649 new cases in 1987—366 are dead
Of the 539 new cases in 1988—213 were dead by 1 January 1989.

(8) Can the AIDS virus be tested for straight away?

You need to have a blood test in order to tell whether or not you have been infected by the AIDS virus, but it takes at least four months after getting the infection for the test to become positive.

(9) Does infection with the AIDS virus last for ever?

Yes. Once you've got the AIDS virus, you have it for the rest of your life.

(10) If you're infected with the AIDS virus, do you get ill immediately?

No. You may be infected with the virus and show no signs of illness for years, maybe in some cases—never. However, even if you are not ill, YOU WILL STILL BE INFECTIOUS TO OTHERS.

(11) Do all people infected with the AIDS virus die from it?

No. At the moment some people who are infected with the virus do not seem to develop the disease, but it is early days yet. However, year by year, of all the people who have the virus infection, gradually more and more develop the disease. Once someone has developed the disease, the chances of dying are very high because at the moment there is no cure.

(12) What are the symptoms?

The first signs of being ill with the AIDS disease can be very vague and very much like other illnesses. Tiredness and swollen glands are common, but having these doesn't mean you've got AIDS. Other symptoms are loss of weight and repeated infections. Whether or not you are worried about having AIDS will depend upon what you have been doing and whether you have put yourself at risk of getting it.

(13) **Is there a cure**?

No. At present there is no cure, and no immediate likelihood of one. Drugs are being tried, which may slow the disease down. Scientists are also working on developing a vaccine to protect against AIDS, but when it is discovered it will take many years to test it.

(14) **Can the AIDS virus be passed on even if you don't know you have it**?

Yes. The blood test only becomes positive several months after the virus has got into the body. Not everyone infected with the virus knows that they've got it, because they won't have had a blood test.

(15) **Where will the virus be in someone who is infected**?

Definitely in: blood, semen, vaginal secretions. It can also be found in: saliva, faeces, tears and urine—but only in very small amounts and it is not thought that you can catch it from them.

It is not found in the skin.

(16) **How can a person catch the AIDS virus**?

Definitely from an infected person by: sharing needles, anal intercourse, an infected mother to her unborn baby, vaginal intercourse. Some people in the past have caught AIDS by being given a blood transfusion with infected blood or infected blood products (including people being treated for haemophilia). But all blood and blood products are now tested, and people who are at high risk of having AIDS are asked not to be blood donors.

You CANNOT catch it by: touching door knobs, sharing dishes and glasses, using lavatory seats, holding hands, having head lice, sneezing and coughing, and swimming in swimming pools.

So far, it is thought that you CANNOT catch it by: kissing or sharing toothbrushes.

(17) **When having sex:**

A man can catch the AIDS virus from an infected man or woman.
A woman can catch it from an infected man.
There are no known cases of a woman catching it from an infected woman.

(18) Groups of people most at risk:

The groups of people most at risk are homosexuals and bisexuals, intravenous drug users, prostitutes; and previously—people having blood transfusions and haemophiliacs. This applies to Britain. However, in certain parts of Africa it is much more a disease of both sexes, and everyone changing sexual partners frequently is at risk. IF YOU AND YOUR PARTNER ONLY HAVE SEX WITH ONE ANOTHER THEN YOU WON'T GET AIDS (unless you are silly enough to use intravenous drugs).

(19) What kills the AIDS virus?

The AIDS virus is very sensitive, and outside the body it doesn't survive very well. It is also killed off by heat, soap and water, and disinfectants. This is why you cannot catch AIDS from an infected person from cups, door knobs and lavatory seats.

(20) Do condoms protect you from catching AIDS?

Yes—almost completely. It is a very good idea to use them always. REMEMBER THEY ALSO PROTECT YOU FROM OTHER SEXUALLY TRANSMITTED DISEASES AND FROM PREGNANCY.

(21) Who can you go to for help?

If you're worried, you ought to talk to someone about your fears. It doesn't really matter who, as long as you find them sympathetic. If you have reason to be really worried, the only way to find out if you are or are not infected with the virus is to have a blood test, and for that you need to see a doctor.

(22) What worries you most?

The survey of your class showed that the top four worries were:
(1) being out of work
(2) a parent or brother or sister dying
(3) failing your exams
(4) not having a 'steady' friend of the opposite sex.
Not surprisingly, this is very different for different people at different times. There is no right or wrong thing to worry about!

Mark (rated by me as only 2/10) seemed to know *all* the answers. Not surprising, seeing what he gets up to. I'd have to be *really* desperate to say 'yes' to him!

Don't think Mum will ever speak to Sal again. We had this discussion about AIDS. I asked Sal about her boy-friends in the last year, and Sal counted on the fingers of both hands—just to get Mum going. Mum went spare. To calm her down, I asked how many boy-friends she'd had before she met Dad. No answer. Just thinking about Mum and Dad doing it turns me off. I wonder what they *actually* got up to before they were married. You'd think they were both totally innocent the way they tell it, and I just don't believe it. Certainly not judging from Mum's old photos Pete found in a box at Aunt Pam's!

9th November

CHARLIE PHONED! He really meant it about not phoning me because he didn't have my number. I'm seeing him next week.

18 Financial Aids

21st November

Missing Pete—much to my surprise. Even the teasing.

My money situation is rather crucial. I don't think I get enough pocket-money, so I did a quick survey of my friends. Poor Kate only gets £1.50—don't know how she manages, but of course she doesn't buy sweets or anything. Mary gets the most. Her parents are divorced too, and she gets £10 a week from her mum AND £10 from her dad. She says she bids them against one another and makes the other one feel guilty. Most of us seem to get around £5, which is what I'm meant to get—when Mum remembers. I used to get this as £20 a month, but would blow it all the first day on a pair of shoes. Mum says it's only for the cinema, presents, tapes, bus fares, make-up and magazines. She buys the clothes and shoes.

Seeing that we work at school, I think we ought to get paid for going there. Then I'd be independent of having to ask Mum all the time. Charlie's working as a garage mechanic apprentice and making £100 a week. Sounded like a fortune till he pointed out that some goes on tax, he pays his mum and dad £25 a week for food and lodging, he has to pay for all his own travel to get to the garage, all his own clothes, AND for taking me to the cinema! I said I'd pay for myself the first time, and then found I couldn't as I didn't have any money. I'm glad he insisted on paying.

I used to be richer when I did baby-sitting, but I've been put off by my experiences. I suppose I could start again, seeing I'm so broke. Or I could get a job like Mary. She works as a glass collector in a wine bar on Saturday and Sunday nights. She gets £5 for two and a half hours. John used to work in the local Wimpy and got £10–12 for six hours. Now he works in a café bar which he hates. He gets £15 for nine hours' work. It's really slave labour and it tires him out.

22nd November

A letter from Pete! Maybe he misses ME!

Dear Susie,

Well, here I am at university. I thought it would be a doddle. But when Mum drove me up, panic set in about ten miles from Nottingham. Will anyone like me? What if no one talks to me? Will they all be cleverer than me? I'm going to drop out. I want a year off.

Mum was great. You know how understanding she can be when she wants. 'You'll be fine, everyone is in the same boat. Just be yourself.' The soundest piece of advice—that.

I got the key to my room, and mail! (Goodness I'm popular, I thought as I filled a carrier bag with a thousand bits of paper.)

The letters all turned out to be about me paying money to join some society or other. My room. Mmmmmh, not bad—small. But I thought a few posters would probably do the trick. I didn't unpack, but went out to find some people to meet. I wasn't going to spend the next five years on my tod. Didn't know a soul. Be American, I kept telling myself. Impose yourself. 'Hi, I'm Pete, how's it going?' 'Have a nice day.' Suddenly it didn't seem so easy, but I've made some friends and I'll tell you all about them when I see you at Christmas.

I'm missing you all, and my room, and you'd better all write to me. Could you send me all the latest football clippings from the back of the local rag? Could you send me my blue pullover from the top drawer in my room (it might need a bit of a wash first), also my other pair of shoes, my folder with the lined paper, and my second pen. And Susie, you have my 'Pot is for Cooking, Not Smoking' tee-shirt. I know I gave it to you but now I want it back. Also my medical dictionary, and my book on 'medical geniuses'. If all this is too much trouble, you could give them all to Sandy who's coming up to see me next week—I hope.

love from your brother

Health Freak Pete

P.S. Sharing a kitchen with a bloke who's managed to create this ideology to defend the fact that he's a lazy bastard. He never cleans up after himself. I'm going to use it when I get back home. P.P.S. Forgot to post this letter when I wrote it five weeks ago! Sorry to hear Bov ate Pinko. I was hoping to experiment on Pinko when I came back at Christmas. You really should have been more careful. (He's a laugh a minute, my brother.)

Pete doesn't know about Charlie yet. Not sure I do really. I had a great time at the cinema last night. No attempted rape!

26th November

AIDS, AIDS, AIDS. Can't see why they call it AIDS when it doesn't aid anyone. Mary says Mini Willie's attitude is, 'I'll have to cut down on the girlies, and if I do have to jump into bed for a bonk then I'll use a johnny, 'cos I can't do without it altogether.'

I don't know one person with AIDS—but had to spend the whole afternoon talking about it at school today. Quite revealing about some of my friends. John said, 'If I caught it, I would try and make the rest of my life more exciting and just as I wanted it. I wouldn't sleep with anybody else so that no one would catch it from me. I don't think I'd tell anyone. I'd probably lose a lot of friends as they'd think I was dirty. I probably would just tell my parents and the person I caught it from, so that they wouldn't give it to anyone else. I think I'd go to a place where other people had AIDS, so I wouldn't feel odd.'

Mary was really awful and said if she caught AIDS, she'd try and give it to as many people as possible and try and take them with her. She said she'd then be so bitter and angry and upset that she'd probably kill herself before kicking the bucket.

While we were talking, a scribbled note was passed from Kate
who sits next to me, saying,

'AIDS advice—don't be silly

Put a condom on your willie.'

As I was laughing, Mr Rogers (of bad breath) found me with it.
He read it, went bright red, and then collapsed trying not to
laugh too.

Emma thought that AIDS had changed her outlook on sex,
and though it wouldn't scare her away from having sex, it would
make her more cautious. She'd be sure to know the person she
was having sex with, and would want to ask her partner about
his previous sex life. She was worried though that he might
think it rude and offensive. Mr Rogers said she shouldn't be
afraid to ask about what other sexual partners someone had
had. It might make all the difference between life and death.
And it wasn't just because of AIDS, but because of all the other
sexually transmitted diseases you could get as well.

I wish the scientists would find a cure for AIDS, because I'm
frightened of catching it when I'm older. People joke about it,
but don't really think about what would happen if they caught it.
I think it's becoming a serious problem in the world, and it's
frightening to think that if you go with someone, you don't know
whether they have got it or not. If I found out that I had AIDS,
and there was an experiment to help find a cure, I'd be willing
to help.

I don't like to see babies on television who have been born
with AIDS. They don't even know that they have it, but they are
going to die. Watching TV programmes about AIDS is really
depressing, because the amount of people who are catching
AIDS is going up. What I didn't like particularly was the
programme about a man who was so angry that he was going to
die from AIDS that he went with everybody he could, so as to
spread the disease. I think that's really selfish—like what Mary
said. Also I watched this serial about a man who caught AIDS.
He had to tell his wife how he'd caught it, by going with a
prostitute. We watched every week and he got worse and worse.
I think this programme must have got across to a lot of people, if
they didn't forget it after a couple of weeks.

'Thought for the Day' written on a toilet wall: 'Last one to get
AIDS is a wanker'.

29th November

I think all is going well with Charlie—at least I hope so. I hardly dare write about it, in case it goes wrong. Sometimes I worry about whether he does fancy me—he's so unpushy.

3rd December

Don't know how Pete manages it—wanting to be a doctor. I think I'd be hopeless. I needed Pete's expertise this morning but it was Sita who knew what to do. We were all outside, between lessons, me avoiding the usual crowd over in one corner smoking fags, when suddenly this boy from the fourth year fell to the ground and started jerking around. I think everyone thought he was joking to begin with, but then a crowd gathered round and just stared. No one knew what to do and we were all getting scared, thinking he was dying or something, when Sita pushed past me and told everyone to stand back and not to touch him and that he'd be all right. I was really impressed. The boy stopped jerking after what seemed ages, but was probably only a minute. Then he seemed to go to sleep. Sita pushed him on to his side, and said this was so that he wouldn't breathe in his sick if he threw up. She said you should do that if someone's had too much to drink as well.

Mr Rogers arrived at this point and sent everyone back into their classrooms—Sita too, which seemed a bit unfair, as she had done everything properly. Afterwards Sita said she had a cousin who used to have fits when he was little, but it only happened when he got a high temperature. Mr Rogers came and said 'thank you' to her later, and explained that the boy had had epilepsy for some time. Normally he didn't have any problems, as long as he took his tablets every morning, but he had forgotten for the last few days.

I think Mr Rogers knew we were all scared because he reassured us that epilepsy only affects about 5 people in every 1,000. With medicines, most people with epilepsy can live perfectly normal lives today, as long as people let them. The worst problem that epileptics have to put up with is other people being frightened of them and treating them as if they are ill all the time, or mental or something. They can do everything everybody else does. They can do jobs, play sports, even swim (as long as they are with somebody).

But it was scary, and I can see how people think epileptics might die when they are having an attack. Mr Rogers said that didn't happen, unless they knocked themselves very hard. He said if you see someone having an attack, all you have to do is to make sure they couldn't hurt themselves against anything. He said that people used to think they should put something into epileptics' mouths to stop them biting their tongue. This is now thought to be wrong, because they might choke on it, or they might bite you by mistake. If you leave them alone, the attack will stop after a few minutes. Then you should do what Sita had done, and lay them on their side, till they wake up. Normally they didn't have to go to hospital or anything, and Sita and I even saw the boy back in the playground in the afternoon. I think he should have said something to Sita, but maybe he didn't know it was her who had helped him, or maybe he was embarrassed. Pete's home next week, so I'll tell him about it.

19 An Itchy and Freaky Christmas

10th December

Pete's home. His usual arrogant self, and a worse 'know all' now he's at university. I think he's still devoted to Sandy, though I'm not so sure the reverse is true. Didn't tell him my suspicions. I do mind for him but I don't want to be the person to have to tell him. I told him all about having to cope with an epileptic fit in school. Nice to be able to tell HIM something for a change.

17th December

Pete's birthday. He's 18! He's not having a party as he had one in Nottingham—with a friend who's also 18 this week. Mum asked if he'd like another one at home, but I think she was rather relieved when he said he'd rather we all went out for a meal.

18th December

Charlie's been away on a training course for two weeks. Now he's back, we're seeing quite a lot of one another. Mum won't let me see him during the week in term time as she thinks it interferes with my work. Mary's mum lets her go out all the time. I sometimes think she doesn't really care about Mary. Although I get angry with Mum, and argue with her about this, actually it's quite good. I can get on with my work and tell Charlie it's all Mum's fault!

All that stuff Pete said about 'sexual sequencing' seems to be true, though I hadn't really considered it before. I thought it was something that only happened to other people, or in books. It never occurred to me during the heat of the action!

I know that Charlie fancies me because he's always looking at me out of the corner of his eye. His hand sometimes brushes against mine as if by accident. He smiles at me a lot, and sits close to me when there are other seats around. He looks at other parts of my body, and he's always nervously checking to see how I respond to what he is saying. Sometimes he even agrees with what I say when I know he really doesn't. I thought only girls did this! He always seems to be licking his lips, which makes me wonder what his expectations are! He has kissed me, but I don't think he's got much experience.

He seemed a bit cool when we first went out. What may have put him off was the way I smelt. Or perhaps my pheromones weren't right. I haven't had a fag in ages, as Charlie did say something about not liking girls who smell like ashtrays. I was wrong about him being into drugs—he's like Pete about that kind of thing.

It must be a nice job researching this 'sexual sequencing' stuff. Better than being a hairdresser for instance (though perhaps that's all to do with sex as well). Sally thinks this science stuff is a load of rubbish and spoils it all anyway.

20th December

Pete's a problem at the moment. Things are not good between him and Sandy. He thinks she's two-timing him. He can't understand what girls are about. Long list of complaints: 'Why can't she say what she wants?' 'Why does she have to keep crying and hinting there's some terrible dark secret?' 'Why did she keep saying she'd tell him about it and then didn't?' He thinks she's trying to tantalize him. Then after being mean to him, she started flirting with him in the pub. She became really angry when Pete rejected her and said she was just doing it because she was drunk. Pete doesn't deserve to be treated like this.

Showed Pete the AIDS questionnaire. He got half the questions wrong, but said it didn't matter as he wasn't in the high risk group. I sometimes wonder.

He has learnt something at medical school about sexually transmitted diseases, though he's not sure how useful some of it would be today. Apparently they used to treat syphilis by applying a roast turnip 'as hot as the patient can bear' to the affected part. I asked, 'What part's that?'

He said that nowadays, if you stick to just one person, then there is virtually no risk of catching AIDS. Five partners a year and you could be spreading to 3,905 people in interrelated contacts over five years. Twenty partners and you're up to three million. Way beyond my maths but obviously not Pete's.

23rd December

Pete's worrying about his health. I think it's all to do with Sandy's dad having died from a heart attack. He was only 56 but smoked twenty a day and 'liked' his food. Pete wants to have the amount of cholesterol in his blood measured. He's sure it must be high. He's heard that most heart attacks are caused by having too much cholesterol in your blood. Apparently almost everybody (70 per cent) has a high cholesterol level in this country compared with America, which is why they think we have more heart attacks than anywhere else in the world. What have they done right in America that we're not doing here? Shouldn't have asked, should I? Not if I didn't want this half-hour lecture.

'*In America they eat wholemeal bread, wholemeal pasta, beans, baked potatoes in their jackets, lentils, brown rice . . .*'

I begged to go to the lav, it was the talk of all this fibre, but the avalanche had begun and wasn't to be turned off. My avalanche would just have to wait.

'. . . *take more regular exercise, drink skimmed milk rather than the full fat stuff, use low fat yoghurt instead of cream, use sunflower spreads instead of butter, cook in polyunsaturated vegetable oil and drain it off the food afterwards, eat more fish, the white bits of the chicken (not the skin), and less red meat . . .*'

Please, please, please I'm bursting!

'. . . *grilled rather than fried food, no chips or sausages, no salt added at the table. We can make do with one-tenth of the salt we eat at the moment.*'

How did he know all these things? He's like a flipping encyclopaedia.

'*It's really up to us. If we buy these things, then the manufacturers will sell them. While we want chips, they'll sell chips. If the NHS is meant to be doing all this preventative stuff, then why isn't the government helping by at least making sure that all school meals are healthy. They must be thinking about it—they've started feeding baked beans to pigs as an experiment to reduce their cholesterol.*'

Just made it to the lav. When I got back, I told him about my success at school with the food questionnaire. Think he was nearly impressed.

Poor Pete, he's got a letter from Sandy and it's all off. Must be why Bov chose today to eat the two goldfish—Leroy and Marvin—that Sandy had given him. Better this way than it just Petering out, ha, ha.

Still off fags.

24th December

Daisy, Paul, and Aunt Jo came for a Christmas tea. They're staying with Aunt Pam so we'll see them again tomorrow. Aunt Jo's getting a divorce. Uncle Geoff's off with his floozie on duty in Northern Ireland. Deserves to get blown up—the way he's treated Aunt Jo.

Pete's found a bit in the paper about boys thinking about sex eight times an hour—on average. He says he thinks about it only once an hour. No doubt for sixty minutes!

25th December

What a Christmas present. Woke up with an itchy bum. Must be worms again. Surely I'm too old to have these. Bet it's from my cousins. I catch everything from them. Dad says you can't get them that quickly. He really is the resident expert on all the nasty things we get. Says human worms come in almost as many varieties as Heinz. Long ones, short ones, thin ones, fat ones, flat ones, hermaphrodite ones. There are worms that travel round your body and lay eggs in mentionable and unmentionable places, ones that make you thin, ones that make your bum itch, ones that are caught from animals, ones that are caught from eating uncooked food, ones that are caught from other human beings—on and on. The commonest one is the thread worm (also known as the pin worm, one of the nematodes or Enterobius vermicularis—but most commonly referred to as just 'the worms') which Dad said was the one I had.

He talks about them as if they were almost friendly! 'They're innocuous little things that inhabit the gut of about one in three of us, most of the time. They come in two sexes—the 'hers' are bigger than the 'hims'—13mm compared with 5mm—and with a diameter of 0.5mm compared with 0.2mm. The poor old pregnant worm is really just made up of two huge wombs—ready to spill out—while all the male has for himself is a curly tail! They mainly live in your gut, near your appendix, and the female creeps out at night to lay her eggs on the skin around your bottom, which is why yours is itching.'

Dad said I'd got worms from someone who'd scratched their own bum because it was itchy. They'd got the eggs under their fingernails, and then touched some food which I'd eaten, so it had all got spread around. Yugh. Don't like the idea that I've eaten something from somebody else's bum. Now they're squirming around inside me having a Christmas feast. Dad says they are easy to get rid of. All I have to do is get some anti-worm medicine, but I can't go to the chemist because they're all closed. The whole family will have to take the medicine—like the anti-louse stuff. It gives your insides a thorough clear-out and gets rid of the worms. But for the next two days, I'm going to have to put up with an itchy bum.

Pete says he's got them too. He wanted to use this as an excuse not to go to Aunt Pam's for lunch. No way Mum was going to let us off though. She said it was up to us, BUT . . . so we had to go. As if going there wasn't bad enough—we even had a lecture from Mum in the car about manners and being nice to Daisy and Paul.

Aunt Pam and Uncle Bob's house was reeking of resident dog shit and cat pee, as usual. I sometimes wonder whether it's always the same turd and piddle that they've never cleared up. There was a four-hour interval before the meal was served up. All jolly Christmas spirit had sunk to zero. What with Uncle Bob being plastered, Gran snoring, Dad with nothing left to say, Mum trying to fill in the ten-minute conversational gaps, Aunt Jo sobbing quietly, Aunt Pam in the kitchen swearing, Daisy reading Aunt Pam's old knitting patterns, Pete and Paul completely disappeared—I just sat and scratched my bum. I think Sal was right to go to her new boy-friend's parents for Christmas. Wish I could have gone with her.

When the meal was finally served, no one could find Pete and Paul. I said they were probably upstairs smoking cannabis and getting high together. Daisy rushed upstairs (I think she wanted to try some too) but found only Dad, smoking a fag. We finally found the boys in the garden playing football. They came in covered with mud and trod more dog shit into the new carpet. Paul tripped over the electric wire to the Christmas tree lights, and the tree fell on to the table. The result was 'needle soup'. Don't think it made it any worse. Aunt Pam definitely wins the Decrepit Aunt's 'Worst Cook of the Year' prize. I'm glad I'm a vegetarian. Uncle Bob's carving was worse than seeing the *Chain-Saw Gang Massacre* on video last week, and Aunt Pam had left the plastic bag of innards inside the turkey. We had the wettest crackers I've ever known. Not one banger worked. Only Aunt Pam and Uncle Bob would wear their paper hats. Everyone else complained that they were too small. I wonder whether they find special morons to write the cracker jokes?

Q. What exams must you sit to become a Farmer?
A. Your Hay-Levels!

Q. What happened to the man who couldn't tell toothpaste from putty?
A. All his windows fell out!

Q. Why did the horse look over the wall?
A. Because he couldn't see through it!

Q. Which would women choose—intelligence or beauty?
A. Beauty, because they know that men aren't intelligent enough to see beyond beauty!

Pete frisked the plum pudding for money, but Aunt Pam's far too mean for that. There was no brandy left to light it, because Uncle Bob had drunk it all. He was so slewed, he even forgot to ask if I'd got a boy-friend yet. The only time I had wanted him to ask, too. Just so I could say, 'Yes'.

Dead silence in the car on the way home. It was even worse than last year. All together, a Very Freaky and Merry Christmas.

Index